THE DIVINE FARMER'S CLASSIC OF MATERIA MEDICA

神農本草經

Shén Nóng Běncǎo Jīng

ALSO BY SABINE WILMS

Venerating the Root:
Sun Simiao's Bei Ji Qian Jin Yao Fang,
volume 5 on Pediatrics • Parts One and Two

Twelve Characters:
A Transmission of Wang Fengyi's Teachings

Let the Radiant Yang Shine Forth:
Lectures on Virtue by Liu Yousheng

THE DIVINE FARMER'S CLASSIC OF MATERIA MEDICA

神農本草經

Shén Nóng Běncǎo Jīng

TRANSLATED BY
SABINE WILMS, PHD

HAPPY GOAT PRODUCTIONS
CORBETT, OREGON • USA

Copyright © 2017 by Sabine Wilms

All rights reserved.
No part of this book may be reproduced in any form
without written permission from the publisher.

PUBLISHED IN THE UNITED STATES OF AMERICA

While the information in this book is given in good faith,
neither the author nor the publisher can be held responsible
for any errors, omissions or use of information contained in
this book. It is imperative that you consult a licensed physician
or other licensed healthcare provider before considering any
of the measures discussed in this publication.

ISBN 978-0-9913429-5-2

Sketches and block prints by Maria Hicks
www.nwfamilyacupuncture.com

Published by Happy Goat Productions
Corbett, Oregon ▪ USA

For more information and to purchase
other works by Sabine Wilms, visit our website:
www.HappyGoatProductions.com

This book

is dedicated to

all humans with dirt under their nails, whether divine or merely mortal, who nurture the earth in harmony with heaven to grow food and medicine that nurture the rest of us,

and

to all the kind souls who write me sweet notes that keep me going! Please continue…

Contents

Table of Illustrations xvi
Foreword xvii
Preface xxv
Acknowledgments xxxvii
Introduction 1
序錄 Preface 13

上藥 Upper Medicinals
草部 Herbs

菖蒲 chāngpú 35
菊花 júhuā 36
人參 rénshēn 38
天門冬 tiānméndōng . . . 39
甘草 gāncǎo 40
乾地黃 gāndìhuáng 42
朮 zhú 43
菟絲子 tùsīzǐ 44
牛膝 niúxī 45
茺蔚子 chōngwèizǐ 46
女萎 nǚwěi 47
防葵 fángkuí 48
柴胡 cháihú 49
麥門冬 màiméndōng . . . 50
獨活 dúhuó 51
車前子 chēqiánzǐ 52

木香 mùxiāng 54
薯蕷 shǔyù 56
薏苡仁 yìyǐrén 57
澤瀉 zéxiè 58
遠志 yuǎnzhì 61
龍膽 lóngdǎn 62
細辛 xìxīn 65
石斛 shíhú 66
巴戟天 bājǐtiān 68
白英 báiyīng 69
白蒿 báihāo 70
赤箭 chìjiàn 71
菴閭子 ānlǘzǐ 72
菥蓂子 xīmíngzǐ 73
蓍實 shīshí 74
赤芝 chìzhī 75

黑芝 hēizhī 76	漏蘆 lòulú 92
青芝 qīngzhī. 77	天名精 tiānmíngjīng . . . 93
白芝 báizhī. 78	決明子 juémíngzi 94
黃芝 huángzhī. 79	飛廉 fēilián 95
紫芝 zǐzhī 80	旋花 xuánhuā 96
卷柏 juǎnbǎi. 81	蘭草 láncǎo 97
藍實 lánshí 82	蛇床子 shéchuángzǐ. . . 98
蘪蕪 míwú. 83	地膚子 dìfūzǐ 99
丹參 dānshēn 84	景天 jǐngtiān 100
絡石 luòshí 85	茵陳蒿 yīnchénhāo . . . 101
蒺藜子 jílízǐ 86	杜若 dùruò 102
肉蓯蓉 ròucōngróng. . . 87	徐長卿 xúchángqīng. . . 103
防風 fángfēng 88	石龍芻 shílóngchú. . . . 104
蒲黃 púhuáng 89	王不留行 wángbùliúxíng . 105
香蒲 xiāngpú 90	升麻 shēngmá 106
續斷 xùduàn. 91	

木部 Trees

牡桂 mǔguì 110	蔓荊實 mànjīngshí. . . 120
菌桂 jūnguì 112	辛夷 xīnyí 121
松脂 sōngzhī. 113	五加皮 wǔjiāpí 122
槐實 huáishí 114	杜仲 dùzhòng 123
枸杞 gǒuqǐ. 115	女貞實 nǚzhēnshí. . . . 124
柏實 bǎishí 116	蕤核 ruíhé 125
茯苓 fúlíng. 117	
榆皮 yúpí 118	
酸棗 suānzǎo 119	

穀部 Food Crops

- 橘柚 *júyòu* 129
- 大棗 *dàzǎo* 130
- 葡萄 *pútáo* 131
- 蓬藟 *pénglěi* 132
- 藕實莖 *ǒushíjīng* 133
- 雞頭實 *jītóushí* 134
- 冬葵子 *dōngkuízǐ* . . . 135
- 莧實 *xiànshí* 136
- 白瓜子 *báiguāzǐ* 137
- 苦菜 *kǔcài* 138
- 胡麻 *húmá* 139

石部 Rocks

- 丹砂 *dānshā* 143
- 雲母 *yúnmǔ* 144
- 玉泉 *yùquán* 145
- 石鐘乳 *shízhōngrǔ* . . 146
- 礬石 *fánshí* 147
- 消石 *xiāoshí* 148
- 朴消 *pòxiāo* 149
- 滑石 *huáshí* 150
- 空青 *kōngqīng* 151
- 曾青 *céngqīng* 152
- 禹餘糧 *yǔyúliáng* . . . 153
- 太一餘糧 *tàiyīyúliáng* . . 154
- 白石英 *báishíyīng* . . . 155
- 紫石英 *zǐshíyīng* 156
- 青石脂 *qīngshízhī* . . . 157
- 赤石脂 *chìshízhī* 158
- 黃石脂 *huángshízhī* . . 159
- 白石脂 *báishízhī* 160
- 黑石脂 *hēishízhī* 161
- 白青 *báiqīng* 162
- 扁青 *biǎnqīng* 163

蟲部 Insects

- 龍骨 *lónggǔ* 166
- 熊脂 *xióngzhī* 168
- 白膠 *báijiāo* 169
- 阿膠 *ējiāo* 170
- 丹雄雞 *dānxióngjī* . . . 171
- 雁肪 *yànfáng* 173
- 石蜜 *shímì* 174
- 蜂子 *fēngzǐ* 175
- 蜜蠟 *mìlà* 176
- 牡蠣 *mǔlì* 177

中藥 MIDDLE MEDICINALS
草部 HERBS

乾薑 gānjiāng 180	白鮮 báixiān 209
葈耳實 xǐěrshí 181	酸漿 suānjiāng 210
葛根 gégēn 182	紫參 zǐshēn 211
栝樓根 guālóugēn . . . 183	藁本 gǎoběn 212
苦參 kǔshēn 184	狗脊 gǒujǐ 213
芎藭 xiōngqióng 185	萆薢 bìxiè 214
當歸 dāngguī 186	白兔藿 báitùhuò 215
麻黃 máhuáng 188	營實 yíngshí 216
通草 tōngcǎo 189	薇銜 wēixián 217
芍藥 sháoyào 191	水萍 shuǐpíng 218
蠡實 líshí 192	王瓜 wángguā 219
瞿麥 qúmài 193	地榆 dìyú 220
玄參 xuánshēn 194	海藻 hǎizǎo 221
秦艽 qínjiāo 195	澤蘭 zélán 222
百合 bǎihé 196	防己 fángjǐ 223
知母 zhīmǔ 197	牡丹 mǔdān 224
貝母 bèimǔ 198	款冬花 kuǎndōnghuā . . 225
白芷 báizhǐ 201	石韋 shíwéi 226
淫羊藿 yínyánghuò . . . 202	馬先蒿 mǎxiānhāo 227
黃芩 huángqín 203	女菀 nǚwǎn 228
石龍芮 shílóngruì . . . 204	王孫 wángsūn 229
茅根 máogēn 205	雲實 yúnshí 230
紫菀 zǐwǎn 206	爵床 juéchuáng 231
紫草 zǐcǎo 207	黃耆 huángqí 232
茜根 qiàngēn 208	黃連 huánglián 234

五味子 wǔwèizǐ 235	姑活 gūhuó 240
沙參 shāshēn 236	屈草 qūcǎo 241
桔梗 jiégěng 237	別羇 biéjī 242
莨蓎子 làngdàngzǐ . . . 238	翹根 qiáogēn 243
陸英 lùyīng 239	萱草 xuāncǎo 244

木部 TREES

梔子 zhīzǐ 246	白棘 báijí 260
竹葉 zhúyè 247	龍眼 lóngyǎn 261
蘗木 bòmù 248	木蘭 mùlán 262
吳茱萸 wúzhūyú 249	桑上寄生 sāngshàngjìshēng . 263
桑根白皮 sānggēnbáipí . 250	柳花 liǔhuā 264
蕪荑 wúyí 252	衛矛 wèimáo 265
枳實 zhǐshí 253	合歡 héhuān 266
厚朴 hòupò 254	松蘿 sōngluó 267
秦皮 qínpí 255	乾漆 gānqī 268
秦椒 qínjiāo 256	石南 shínán 269
山茱萸 shānzhūyú . . . 257	蔓椒 mànjiāo 270
紫葳 zǐwēi 258	欒華 luánhuá 271
豬苓 zhūlíng 259	淮木 huáimù 272

穀部 FOOD CROPS

梅實 méishí 274	水斳 shuǐqín 279
蓼實 liǎoshí 275	粟米 sùmǐ 280
葱實 cōngshí 276	黍米 shǔmǐ 281
水蘇 shuǐsū 277	麻蕡 máfén 282
瓜蔕 guādì 278	

石部 ROCKS 283

石硫黃 shíliúhuáng . . . 284	理石 lǐshí 288
石膏 shígāo 285	長石 chángshí 289
磁石 císhí 286	孔公孽 kǒnggōngniè . . . 290
陽起石 yángqǐshí 287	殷孽 yīnniè 291

蟲部 INSECTS

髮髲 fàbì 294	伏翼 fúyì 303
白馬莖 báimǎjīng 295	鱧魚 lí or luǒyú 304
鹿茸 lùróng 296	鯉魚膽 lǐyúdǎn 305
羖羊角 gǔyángjiǎo 297	烏賊魚骨 wūzéiyúgǔ . . 306
牡狗陰莖 mǔgǒuyīnjīng 298	海蛤 hǎigé 307
羚羊角 língyángjiǎo . . . 299	石龍子 shílóngzǐ 308
牛黃 niúhuáng 300	白僵蠶 báijiāngcán . . . 309
麝香 shèxiāng 301	桑螵蛸 sāngpíxiāo 310
天鼠屎 tiānshǔshǐ 302	

下藥 LOWER MEDICINALS
草部 HERBS

附子 fùzǐ 312	草蒿 cǎohāo 320
烏頭 wūtóu 313	旋覆花 xuánfùhuā 321
天雄 tiānxióng 314	藜蘆 lílú 322
半夏 bànxià 315	鉤吻 gōuwěn 323
虎掌 hǔzhǎng 316	射干 shègān 324
鳶尾 yuānwěi 317	蛇含 shéhán 325
大黃 dàhuáng 318	恆山 héngshān 326
葶藶 tínglì 319	蜀漆 shǔqī 327

甘遂 gānsuì 328
白蘞 báiliǎn 329
青葙子 qīngxiāngzǐ . . . 330
雚菌 guànjūn 331
白及 báijí 332
大戟 dàjǐ 333
澤漆 zéqī 334
茵芋 yīnyù 335
貫眾 guànzhòng 336
蕘花 yáohuā / ráohuā . . 337
牙子 yázǐ 338
羊躑躅 yángzhízhú . . . 339
芫花 yuánhuā 340
商陸 shānglù 341
羊蹄 yángtí 342
萹蓄 biānxù 343
狼毒 lángdú 344
鬼臼 guǐjiù 345

白頭翁 báitóuwēng . . . 346
羊桃 yángtáo 347
女青 nǚqīng 348
連翹 liánqiáo 349
石下長卿 shíxiàchángqīng . 350
蘭茹 lǔrú 351
烏韭 wūjiǔ 352
鹿藿 lùhuò 353
蚤休 zǎoxiū 354
石長生 shícháng shēng . . 355
藎草 jìncǎo 356
牛扁 niúbiǎn 357
夏枯草 xiàkūcǎo 358
敗醬 bàijiàng 359
白薇 báiwēi 360
積雪草 jīxuěcǎo 361
蜀羊泉 shǔyángquán . . 362

木部 TREES

巴豆 bādòu 364
蜀椒 shǔjiāo 365
皂莢 zàojiá 366
楝實 liànshí 367
鬱李仁 yùlǐrén 368
莽草 mǎngcǎo 369
雷丸 léiwán 370

梓白皮 zǐbáipí 371
桐葉 tóngyè 372
藥實根 yàoshígēn . . . 373
黃環 huánghuán 374
溲疏 sōushū 375
鼠李 shǔlǐ 376

穀部 Food Crops

桃核仁 táohérén 378	苦瓠 kǔhù 382
杏核仁 xìnghérén 380	大豆黃卷 dàdòuhuángjuǎn . 383
假蘇 jiǎsū 381	腐婢 fǔbì 384

石部 Rocks

石膽 shídǎn 386	粉錫 fěnxī 395
雄黃 xiónghuáng 388	代赭 dàizhě 396
雌黃 cíhuáng 389	鹵鹹 lǔxián 397
水銀 shuǐyín 390	青琅玕 qīnglánggān . . . 399
膚青 fūqīng 391	礜石 yùshí 400
凝水石 níngshuǐshí . . . 392	石灰 shíhuī 401
鐵落 tiěluò 393	白堊 báiè 402
鉛丹 qiāndān 394	冬灰 dōnghuī 403

蟲部 Insects

六畜毛蹄甲 liùchùmáotíjiǎ . 406	馬刀 mǎdāo 417
豚卵 túnluǎn 407	蟹 xiè 418
麋脂 mízhī 408	蛇蛻 shétuì 419
鼺鼠 léishǔ 409	蝟皮 wèipí 420
燕屎 yànshǐ 410	蠮螉 yēwēng 421
龜甲 guījiǎ 411	蜣蜋 qiāngláng 422
蝦蟆 hámá 412	蛞蝓 kuòyú 423
鮀魚甲 tuóyújiǎ 413	白頸蚯蚓 báijǐngqiūyǐn . 424
鱉甲 biējiǎ 414	蠐螬 qícáo 425
蚱蟬 zhàchán 415	石蠶 shícán 426
露蜂房 lúfēngfáng . . . 416	雀甕 quèwèng 427

樗雞 chūjī 428	鼠婦 shǔfù 436
斑蝥 bānmáo 429	水蛭 shuǐzhì 437
螻蛄 lóugū 430	木虻 mùméng 438
蜈蚣 wúgōng 431	蜚虻 fěiméng 439
馬陸 mǎlù 432	蜚蠊 fěilián 440
地膽 dìdǎn 433	䗪蟲 zhèchóng 441
螢火 yínghuǒ 434	貝子 bèizǐ 442
衣魚 yīyú 435	彼子 bǐzǐ 443

上藥 Upper Medicinals · Notes   445
中藥 Middle Medicinals · Notes   453
下藥 Lower Medicinals · Notes   465

Glossary   485
Bibliography   503
Medicinals Index – Pinyin   507
Medicinals Index – Latin   515
Medicinals Index – English   523
Cross-Reference List for Modern Medicinal
  Pinyin Names   529
General Index   531

Table of Illustrations

Block Print 1 - *gāncǎo*   41
Block Print 2 - *guìzhī*   111
Block Print 3 - *sháoyào*   190

Sketch 1 - *júhuā*   37
Sketch 2 - *chēqiánzǐ*   53
Sketch 3 - *mùxiāng*   55
Sketch 4 - *zéxiè*   59
Sketch 5 - *yuǎnzhì*   60
Sketch 6 - *lóngdǎn*   63
Sketch 7 - *xìxīn*   64
Sketch 8 - *shíhú*   67
Sketch 9 - *shēngmá*   107
Sketch 10 - *dāngguī*   187
Sketch 11 - *báizhǐ*   200
Sketch 12 - *huángqí*   233

Foreword

by E. N. Anderson

The *Divine Farmer's Classic of Materia Medica* is the earliest surviving herbal in the Chinese medical tradition. It dates from the Eastern (or Later) Han Dynasty, around 100–200 CE. The name refers to China's ancient god of farming and medicine, supposedly a minister of agriculture under the mythical Yellow Emperor in the 28th–29th centuries BCE. The book's title was never intended to suggest that Shén Nóng actually *wrote* the book, only that it consisted of lore going back to him in some sense (mythical if not literal). However, this book and other early works were later ascribed to his authorship, and this is the source of the claim, still seen occasionally, that "the Chinese" were writing about sagebrush or soybeans or some other crop over a millennium before they had a writing system. The actual compilers of the *Divine Farmer's Classic* are not known. They were almost certainly medical men, and they wrote during the latter part of the Han Dynasty (206 BCE – 220 CE).

Originally containing 365 medicinals—one for each day of the year—the book has been substantially edited, damaged, re-created, commented on, and otherwise transformed throughout Chinese history. The major work of restoring and editing it was done by the great Daoist religious thinker and medical expert Tao Hongjing (ca. 456 – 536) in the 6th century CE.

For centuries, this book was all the world knew of ancient Chinese herbal lore. However, in the last century, a trickle of archaeologically recovered herbal documents has confirmed and somewhat extended our knowledge. In particular, bamboo slips found in a tomb at Mawangdui in 1973 contain a large part of an earlier herbal work. About half the herbs mentioned there are in the *Shén Nóng Běncǎo Jīng* (Unschuld 1986:15). It is probably safe to say that this work incorporated all the best knowledge available in Chinese medical circles in the 2nd century CE.

Běncǎo literally means "basic herbal." *Jīng* literally means a warp book, with reference to the warp threads on a loom—the basic threads that give the whole structure and foundation to the cloth. (The cross-running "weft" books are the commentaries and secondary literature on the true classics, the "warps.") Thus a *jīng* is not necessarily a literary classic; it is a foundational work for a field. Such is the present book—it is the true foundation of Chinese herbal science. And science it truly is; it is singularly free from, on the one hand, the demons and spirits of Chinese magical lore, and, on the other, the artificial and speculative systemic correspondences that dominated much of Han Dynasty elite medicine. The present book records only known or inferred values of the medicinal substances in question.

In many cases, the values of these medicines are real and substantial. In others, the values are now hard to demonstrate; often, they were inferred on the basis of hope, confirmation bias, or placebo effect. Unfortunately, most of the plants are so little studied, and the illness terms are so hard to equate with modern ones, that we cannot know. Unfortunately, we have very little idea of what the names of illnesses signified in China 2000 years ago. "Running piglet," for one rather striking example, referred to some condition that felt as if a piglet were running around inside the body—possibly rapidly ascending and descending energies; we will never know. On the plant, animal, and mineral names, we have better control, since those tombs that contained medical texts often contained the medicines too, with labels that show word usage has not changed much (if at all).

One must remember—here as with other herbals, and, for that matter, modern drugs—that a very slight effect was better than nothing. Societies lacking modern antibiotics treasured anything that would produce any benefit at all.

The medicinal knowledge here is the start of a real scientific tradition. It is not perfect. It requires qualification on the basis of present knowledge. But it is a genuine attempt to create a systematic, empirical medicine, theorized as well as one could theorize herbal knowledge in the 2nd century. The basic theoretical construct is the flow of *qì*, the subtle energies and substances whose circulation in the body and the cosmos produce life and flux. It could be disrupted by many factors, and often a cure was considered to work by normalizing the flows and proportions of various forms of *qì*. This observational and theoretical approach is identified with scholarly Daoism.

Arrangement of drugs institutionalized a division into upper-level drugs that function as rulers, mid-level drugs that function as vassals or ministers, and lower-level ones that act as assistants and messengers. (The word generally translated as "rulers" actually means "gentlemen," "members of the elite," but has always been taken to mean sovereign drugs.) The upper drugs are those that have a general tonic or strengthening or life-protecting effect, such as ginseng. Most of them remain central to Chinese medicine today. The middle drugs are more directly active, with some degree of visible or sensible physiological effect. Several of these drugs have clear and well-known physical action, others remain inadequately studied.

The lowest level are drugs that are described as "having poison." (Upper drugs lack it.) They have direct medical effects, often actual toxins. They are often bactericidal and fungicidal, or otherwise obviously effective, but dangerous to the taker also. These include aconite, henbane, sagebrush, false hellebore, and other frankly toxic plants, but also items like lepidium and smartweed that have a strong, peppery effect on the mouth but no actual poison. The Chinese medical term *dú* 毒 "poison" does not necessarily mean that an item is poisonous itself; it may merely potentiate poisons already in the system, thus worsening illness. In western terms, it is these lower-class drugs that are the "effective" ones, but analysis of the higher-level ones has scarcely begun (in most cases), and we do not really understand their subtle overall effects.

After Tao Hongjing edited and commented on the *Shén Nóng Běncǎo Jīng* (his commentaries and additions are not included here), the *bencao* literature grew and propagated. Dozens of herbals appeared, including specialized ones on foreign herbs, southern herbs, and so on. The literature climaxed in Li Shizhen's definitive

Běncǎo Gāng Mù of 1596, now available in English in six huge volumes (Li 2003).

It is interesting to compare the Chinese herbal tradition with the one developing at the same time in the west. Theophrastus, writing in the 4th century BCE in Greece, put botany on a scientific footing before China was known to have equivalent works. However, the first great western herbal, that of Pedanius Dioscorides, was almost exactly contemporary with the *Shén Nóng Běncǎo Jīng*. It is also similar in size and method of description. Dioscorides and Galen developed a scientific approach, free of magic and of excessive systematization, and thus quite comparable to that of Shén Nóng's herbal.

Western herbals developed more or less in step with the Chinese, climaxing in the enormous and extremely thorough compilations of Al-Bīrūnī and Avicenna, building on the work of Galen and Dioscorides, in Central Asia in the 11th century. It is no accident that these two brilliant men were writing at the very center of the Silk Road. At this time, that route was the main corridor for intellectual exchange between east and west. The two Muslims show some, but only slight, knowledge of east Asian medicine, but the flow from west to east was more substantial, and under the Mongols it reached a climax, with great works appearing in China that summarized western medicine for Chinese benefit.

Herbal knowledge rose to new heights in Renaissance Europe. The herbals of Rembert Dodoens and others brought herbal lore into early modern science at exactly the same time that Li Shizhen was working on his definitive book. Dodoens' main herbal appeared in 1554, and was strikingly similar in coverage, size, approach, and scientific insight to Li's. But after that, the long parallel development was broken. China collapsed into wars, from which emerged the Qing Dynasty, a highly conservative age that did not stimulate much new development. Li remains the standard of Chinese medicinal tradition.

Sabine Wilms has now provided a rigorous translation and bilingual edition of this first of China's surviving herbals. The *Shén Nóng Běncǎo Jīng* has been enormously important historically, and is still the basis for a great deal of traditional Chinese herbal practice. This translation makes the text available with a fine analytic rendering into English.

Sabine Wilms' edition is rigorous, carefully done, and designed to be maximally useful. Plant identifications are according to the best current science, including recent taxonomic revisions. Medical terms follow recent best usage. This book will bring China's first herbal to an English-speaking audience, and also provide correct scientific names and valuable scholarly annotations to all readers and users of the book. A classic work that has been used for almost two thousand years is getting yet another revival and yet another new life.

Books cited:

Li Shizhen. 2003. Compendium of Materia Medica (Bencao Gangmu). Tr. Xiao Xiaoming, Li Zhenguo, and committee. Chinese original 1596. Beijing: Foreign Languages Press.

Unschuld, Paul. 1986. Medicine in China: A History of Pharmaceutics. Berkeley: University of California Press.

Preface

by Sabine Wilms, PhD

夫為醫者，再讀醫書耳。讀而不能為醫者有矣，未有不讀而能為醫者也。

Physicians undoubtedly immerse themselves in the medical texts! People who study [the texts] but are incapable of practicing as physicians certainly do exist. But there has never been anybody who does not study and yet is capable of practicing as a physician.

Southern Sòng History,
preface to the *Líng Shū* 靈樞 "Divine Pivot"

No tree, it is said, can grow to heaven unless its roots reach down to hell.

C.G. Jung, *Aion: Researches into the Phenomenology of the Self*, 1951

It is not just because I am a farmer with dirt under my nails that the "Divine Farmer's Classic of Materia Medica" has always been one of my favorite books.

As a critical historian and teacher of classical Chinese medicine at the National University of Natural Medicine and elsewhere, I firmly believe this little book to be one of the most important, foundational texts of this medicine that I love so dearly and have dedicated my life to. For this reason, Happy Goats Productions has decided to produce a literal and clean translation, with the earliest currently available Chinese source text side-by-side with my English rendition.

Our intention is two-fold: On the one hand, we want those of you with no access to a solid edition of the Chinese source text or no ability to read classical Chinese on their own to enjoy this gem with as little outside interpretation or alteration as possible. For this reason I have chosen a faithful and very literal translation of the text over an elegant and perhaps more easily digestible interpretation. On the other hand, we hope that the bilingual layout encourages those of you who possess some background in classical Chinese to look at the Chinese text while reading my translation, so that you can gain a deeper understanding of the text than any translation could ever offer.

After decades of struggling with translating philosophical, cosmological, and medical literature from classical Chinese to English, I have come to the conclusion that no translation could ever do justice to the depth of the original source. The gap between early

Chinese and modern English culture is simply too large to find direct equivalents for too many terms and phrases, from qì to *shén* ("spirit(s)," if you must give it an English word). Moreover, any translation will always by necessity be limited by the translator's own level of cultivation and understanding of the material, and when it comes to the pursuit of immortality or harmony between Heaven and Earth, we modern people are not even scratching the surface of what the ancient texts have to offer us. For this reason, I encourage all my readers to make friends with the Chinese part of the text as well, to engage with it in whatever way you can, to write it out in calligraphy, have a native speaker read it out loud for you, run it through a Chinese translation software, memorize it, sleep on it, or read it to your dog. For many entries, the grammar patterns are not that difficult and quite repetitive. For this reason, this book is actually an ideal text to study classical Chinese with, especially if you are a practitioner of Chinese medicine. May this book encourage you to dip your toes in the "bubbling spring" (湧泉, *yǒngquán*, a.k.a. KI-1) of the medical classics so that they become a frequently-visited source of rejuvenation and joy for yourself and of inspiration and clarity for your clinical practice.

Whether you are a practicing physician or pharmacist, a fellow "herb head" and plant lover, a historian of early Chinese culture and natural science, or just curious about one of the most ancient texts from early Chinese literature, we sincerely hope that you will enjoy this text as much as we do!

One reason for the importance of this text is obviously the ancient origin of the knowledge contained therein and its association with *Shén Nóng*, a name that translates literally as "Divine Farmer." This ancient semi-mythological culture hero of Chinese civilization has been celebrated for thousands of years in China for the invention of agriculture, among many other achievements. A text from the second century BCE called *Huáinánzǐ* 淮南子 recounts the following legend:

古者，民茹草飲水，采樹木之實，食蠃蠬之肉。時多疾病毒傷之害，於是神農乃始教民播種五穀，相土地宜，燥濕肥墝高下，嘗百草之滋味，水泉之甘苦，令民知所辟就。當此之時，一日而遇七十毒。

In ancient times, the people subsisted on grasses to eat and water to drink, picked fruits and nuts from the trees and ate the meat of snails and clams. They frequently fell ill due to being injured by poisoning. For this reason the Divine Farmer began to teach the people how to sow and cultivate the Five Grains and assess the suitability of land and soil for dryness and moistness, fertile or rocky ground, and high or low elevation. He tasted the flavors of the hundred herbs and sweetness and bitterness of the water in their springs, letting the people know what places to avoid and what places to draw near to. During this time, he encountered seventy poisons in a single day.

In addition to his association with agriculture, bibliographic records and citations from the Han dynasty on connect Shén Nóng's name to titles on the subject of "nurturing life" (養生 *yǎng shēng*), or in other words, the prevention of illness and preservation and optimization of health for the purpose of prolonging one's lifespan or even attaining immortality by transcending the limitations of the mortal body. The content as well as the value judgments inherent in the categorization of medicinals in this text will show the astute reader the significance of this association with a tradition not primarily concerned with treating illness but with preventing it and with promoting longevity or even immortality instead. It is no coincidence either that the single other key figure associated with the *Běncǎo Jīng*, namely the historical figure Táo Hóngjǐng (see below), is better known in Chinese history as the founder of the Shàngqīng 上清 ("Supreme Clarity") school of Daoism. His biography aptly depicts him as a hermit who specialized in academic, religious, and alchemical research into methods of transcending the limitations of the natural human body by transforming it into a refined immortal existence, similar to the emergence of a butterfly from the chrysalis.

Materia medica literature, called 本草 *běncǎo* ("roots and grasses") in Chinese, has a long and illustrious, if somewhat overwhelming, history in Chinese medicine. The trusted catalogue of Chinese medical literature *Zhōngguó Yī Jí Kǎo* 中國醫籍考 ("Investigation of Chinese Medical Literature"), published in 1819 by the Japanese scholar Tanba no Mototane, lists no fewer than 2,605 titles, a number that does not include the subsequent category of *shízhì* 食治 ("Materia Dietetica").[1] In Mototane's work, the title *Shén Nóng Běncǎo Jīng* ("Divine Farmer's Classic of Materia Medica") appears as the first book in the category of *běncǎo* 本草 ("materia medica"). Although recorded as a text in three volumes in the bibliography of the Sui 隨 Dynasty (581-618 CE), the original, if we can even speak of a single source at all, has unfortunately not survived. Due to later scholars' respect for the information contained in this work, however, we have countless copies of the preface and the text of the individual entries, as quoted in the major materia medica literature from classical times on. With some minor disagreements on the placement and order of individual substances in

---

1 I gratefully accept the count by Paul U. Unschuld in his Medicine in China. A History of Pharmaceutics, p. 2.

one or the other of the three categories, scholars agree that the original text contained descriptions of 365 medicinal substances, classified into the three categories of "upper," "middle," and "lower" in accordance with their effect on the human body and their association with Heaven, Humanity, and Earth, respectively.

The preservation of this treasure trove of early Chinese knowledge about the natural world may be due mostly to the efforts of one of the earliest and most illustrious proponents of this text: the abovementioned scholar, author, and Daoist practitioner Táo Hóngjǐng 陶弘景 (452–536), style name Yǐn Jū 隱居 ("Living in Hiding").

As Táo's preface to the text shows, it was already obvious to scholars in the early sixth century that the information contained in the various materia medica texts associated with the Divine Farmer did not come directly from his pen but had been expanded on in the process of oral transmission over thousands of years:

> 舊說皆稱《神農本草經》，余以為信然。昔神農氏之王天下也畫易卦以通鬼神之情;造耕種以省煞害之弊;宣藥療疾，以拯夭傷之命。此三道者，歷群聖而滋彰。文王、孔子，象象繫辭，幽贊人天。后稷、伊尹，播厥百谷，惠被生民。岐、皇、彭、扁，振揚輔導，恩流含氣。並歲逾三千，民到於今賴之。但軒轅以前，文字未傳，如六爻指垂，畫象稼穡。。。

The old explanations all refer to a *"Divine Farmer's Classic of Materia Medica."* I consider this to be reliable. In the past, in his rule of Under Heaven, the Divine Farmer drew the trigrams of the "Classic of Changes" to provide access to the dispositions of the supernatural entities; set up the plowing and planting of fields to save people from death from terminal injuries; and promulgated [information on] medicinals and the curing of illnesses, to rescue from the fate of premature loss of life and damages. These three Teachings (lit. "Dao") were [then] enriched and illuminated by passing through large numbers of sages. King Wén and Confucius added judgments, images, and commentaries, acclaiming humanity and heaven through obscurity. Hòu Jì and Yī Yǐn disseminated the Hundred Grains, bestowing their benevolence on all living people. Qí Bó, Huángdì, Péngzǔ, and Biǎn Què provided guidance and support with great fervor. In this way, the [Divine Farmer's] beneficence has circulated and remained alive. And even though three thousand years have gone by, the people still rely on it to this day!

Nevertheless, before the time of the Yellow Emperor, written characters were not yet transmitted and the six lines [from the Classic of Changes] were bequeathed to posterity with finger gestures, while the tasks of sowing and reaping were transmitted by means of pictures…

While in pursuit of immortality, alchemical transformation of the body, and transcendence of this mundane world in his hermitage on Mount Máo, Táo Hóngjǐng collated and compiled the materia medica information of his times into first a shorter three-volume, and then a longer seven-volume version of a so-called "Classic of Materia Medica." Making matters a bit confusing, he titled the first one *Shén Nóng Běncǎo Jīng* 神農本草經 ("Divine Farmer's Classic of Materia Medica") and the second one *Běncǎo Jīng Jí Zhù* 本草經集註 ("Collected Comments on the Classic of Materia Medica"). Their content overlaps substantially, and these texts have themselves been lost in their original version. Nevertheless, because the text of Táo's materia medica, regardless of the version, has been quoted and expanded on innumerable times by later authors, it has been possible to reconstruct the original with considerable confidence.

In his preface to the "Collected Comments," Táo mentions that the original information of the text, referred to by its abbreviated title as *Běn Jīng* 本經 ("Root Classic"), was first written down during the Hàn dynasty in four volumes, one containing general information and the other three containing monographs on medicinal substances in three categories associated with Heaven, Humanity, and Earth respectively. Táo further explains that his work includes an expansion of the original 365 substances by another 365 substances and commentaries by himself and by "famous physicians" (名醫 *míng yī*) on such topics as alternate names, information on growing, harvesting, preparation, and storage, and medicinal uses, which he set off from the original text by using a different ink color. Táo's collected commentaries were subsequently published separately under the title *Míng Yī Bié Lù* 名醫別錄 ("Separate Records by Famous Physicians"). More importantly, however, the text of his original "Classic of Materia Medica" and the commentary by himself and the "Famous Doctors" has been preserved and expanded upon ever since, ensuring not just their survival but their continued preponderance as one of the pivotal texts in the traditional literature of Chinese medicine.

In contemporary Chinese bookstores, editions of the *Shén Nóng Běncǎo Jīng* are ubiquitous but unfortunately not consistent in regards to the order, numbering, and classification of substances. This does not need to concern the practitioner who is merely looking for information contained in the individual monographs. It can, however, cause serious headaches to critical scholars or translators like myself who are trying to publish a new version of the text. Táo Hóngjǐng himself had already mentioned categorizing the monographs both in the original three tiers of upper, middle, and lower, and in accordance with their natural origin into "precious stones" (玉石 *yù shí*), "herbs and trees" (草木 *cǎo mù*), "insects and wild animals" (蟲獸 *chóng shòu*) and "fruits, vegetables, rice, and grains" (果菜米穀 *guǒ cài mǐ gǔ*), as most scholars believe he had done in his own edition. At this particular moment, I have more than a dozen Chinese versions of this text in front of me, all called *"Shén Nóng Běncǎo Jīng"* and claiming to be critical historical editions. Hardly any of them agree with one another on the precise number, classification, and arrangement of the monographs. For the purposes of this book, I have chosen to follow the arrangement suggested by the eminent researcher of early classical medical literature Mǎ Jìxìng 馬繼興 in his new critical edition from 2012, because I have complete faith in his lifetime of research into the textual history of China's medical classics (he was born in 1925!).

While I would have loved to spend weeks researching each single substance and could have compiled dozens of pages on the various commentaries to each entry, I have decided to limit the content of this edition strictly to what is believed to have been the earliest layer of the text. Wanting to let the ancient classic speak for itself as faithfully to the original as possible in an affordable and manageable modern English edition, I have even refrained from including Táo Hóngjǐng's commentary. There is always time for another book in the future…

Acknowledgments

by Sabine Wilms, PhD

Translating a text associated with as lofty a figure as the "Divine Farmer" is no small task. As a result, the book you are holding in your hands is already the third edition, within less than a year of its publication. From my initial translation work more than two dozen years ago until now, more people have helped generously with this project than I will ever be able to recall, and this book would have never come to fruition without them.

My love affair with this text began when I was compiling a materia medica index for my doctoral dissertation on the writings on gynecology by Sūn Sīmiǎo 孫思邈. I translated the entries on specific medicinals in the *Shén Nóng Běncǎo Jīng* as part of my effort to understand the intended effect of gynecological formulas on suffering female bodies, to learn more about early Chinese gynecological etiology, pathology, and treatment. My ability to both understand and contextualize early Chinese texts of any genre, but of philosophical, religious, scientific, and cosmological content in particular, has benefited immensely from the strict guidance I received from my dissertation advisor at the University of Arizona, Dr. Donald Harper. Also at the University of Arizona, Dr. Mark Nichter introduced me to the wonderful world of medical anthropology by teaching me how to ask the right questions in discourses on medicine, healing, and the body, a skill that I am refining with gusto to this day. Following graduation, I was fortunate to work closely for two years with Dr. Nigel Wiseman in my position as translator for Paradigm Publications. I owe my sensitivity to issues of technical terminology and English translation of Chinese medical literature for practitioners to his unrelenting feedback.

In terms of my clinical understanding, I have benefited from countless conversations with countless colleagues, friends, and students all over the world over the past two decades. Thank you all from the bottom of my heart for always so patiently answering my questions, for providing such essential critical feedback, for allowing me to be a fly on the wall and sit in on your classes and conversations, and for reminding me of the clinical relevance of my work. I consider myself so fortunate, as an academic and translator of "ancient" historical material, to have an audience of people who care so deeply about the wisdom in the early Chinese texts and therefore about my work, because they are convinced that it affects their ability to alleviate the suffering of their patients in their daily practice. What more could a historian ask for! As it is impossible here to list all the people who have contributed to my understanding of Chinese medicine as a living practice, I limit myself to two of my colleagues at the College of Classical Chinese Medicine at the National University of Natural Medicine who have taught me so much in the recent past: Dr. Long Rihui and Dr. Brenda Hood. I cannot thank you enough for your patience and generosity in answering my questions, but more importantly for embodying the true "eminent physician" as envisioned by Sūn Sīmiǎo in the way you conduct your daily life.

Most instrumental for the editing and review of my initial manuscript have been Leo Lok, practitioner of Chinese medicine and independent scholar of classical Chinese medical literature, and medical anthropologist Dr. Eugene Anderson, who both took precious time out of their busy schedules to review my lengthy manuscript entry by entry. They spotted errors and inconsistencies, added additional information and insights, and asked questions that forced me to revise or clarify translations and compose more explanatory footnotes. As a single mother, I know that it does take a village to raise a child (and helpful neighbors to keep a herd of goats in production). Likewise, I have learned through decades of publishing work that the quality of a book truly does depend on a team of trained professionals, especially when it involves a translation from classical Chinese. This book has benefited immensely from just such a team and would not have happened without it.

Since its first publication almost exactly a year ago, this book has gone through a number of additions and corrections. I sincerely hope that I will finally be able to put this project to rest and move on to other topics once the final manuscript for this third edition is submitted to the printer... at least until the artist Maria Hicks completes more woodblock prints and sketches so that we can get to work on a three-volume boxed-set edition. Many of the changes to this third edition, such as a corrected tone in the pinyin for an alternate medicinal name based on the likely meaning of the character in my translation, will not be apparent or even relevant to any but the most discerning reader. Nevertheless, this book aims and claims to be the most academically solid and reliable translation of one of the most important classics in Chinese medicine and as such to serve as the go-to reference for any practitioner or scholar who needs access to its contents in a Western language. Based on the responsibility of this intention, I have involved a number of additional helpers in this edition to bring this book that much closer to that goal. Here are the major changes in a nutshell:

The improvements in the cover design and especially in the interior layout throughout the translated text are the wonderful work of Barbara Tada, who has finally allowed this book to become the visible manifestation of my internal vision that I have carried inside me for a number of years. I could not be happier with the outcome!

Meg Chuang, a current dual-degree doctoral candidate at the National University of Natural Medicine, has poured over every single character and pinyin pronunciation with her formidable hawk eyes and thereby assured the highest possible degree of accuracy and consistency between the Chinese characters, the pinyin pronunciation, and the English translation. With her clinical expertise in Chinese medicine, classical texts training, and dual Chinese and English language background, she is the editor and proof-reader that every other publisher in the field of Chinese medicine can only dream of.

Justin Penoyer has kindly allowed me to share a cross-reference list he created for contemporary pinyin medicinal names where these differ from the names in the original text. In addition, I have added a few more footnotes and Glossary entries for diseases in response to questions and feedback from readers.

Like all other books here at Happy Goat Productions, the person most affected by this labor of love has been my daughter Momo who has often dragged me away from my computer to eat or sleep. With the assistance of happy dogs and goats, she has kept me rooted in the real world. No words can ever be enough to express the gratitude I feel for her presence in my life.

Lastly, Happy Goat Productions would not even exist without all the support and encouragement I continue to receive from readers, students, and colleagues. You have made all the difference, whether by buying and reading my books, by sending sweet notes, encouraging feedback, and wonderful critical questions, or perhaps most importantly for such a small business, by spreading the word about my books. Your support and interest gives me the persistence and strength to keep on writing and publishing.

Introduction

1. The Problem With Medicinal Identification

To improve the reader's understanding of the content of this book through a more intuitive and sensory access to the substances discussed therein, we have included the following information for each entry: After the Chinese text you will find

- the pinyin pronunciation, which is how Chinese medicinals are referred to in the clinical context of contemporary Chinese Medicine,

- a literal translation of the Chinese characters in quotation marks, when these contain any potentially meaningful information at all. In instances where characters are used purely for phonetic reasons and no semantic connection could be established, this information is missing.

- the scientific identification, including the specific part of the plant or animal used, whenever possible, and

- an English common name in parentheses, whenever applicable. Please note that this information is given with some hesitation, to give the reader a very general sense of the substance discussed but not to aid in identification. These common names often refer to plant families instead of a specific species, and we therefore cannot assume that a local variety would have the same medicinal effect as described in this text.

Please note that this translation is not a scientific treatise and that I am a translator of early Chinese medical literature, not a specialist in pharmaceutical identification. Moreover, the exact and unequivocal equation of ancient Chinese terms with modern substances is often far from certain, if not impossible. Like in any other medical tradition worldwide, the problems of identification and local variation have been debated by Chinese scholars, practitioners, scientists, wildcrafters, growers, pharmacists, and other "plant people" since the time of the Divine Farmer. Before you use any substance on the basis of the English identification in this work, please consult the pertinent medical and scientific literature and seek the advice of trained professionals. For the purpose of the present book, I have tended to select general English terms that may give the reader some insight into the type of substance discussed, based on her or his familiarity with perhaps a more common variety, but these terms often refer to many different species depending on the area of the world you might live in. Whether a particular local species or variety might serve as an appropriate substitution for medicinal usage is not a question this book is attempting to address.

Whenever scholarly consensus has been able to ascertain the common identity over distances of time and space, the botanical identifications found in this book are based on the 1982 edition of the *Zhōngyào Dà Cídiǎn* 中藥大辭典 ("Great Dictionary of Chinese Medicinals"). Dr. Eugene Anderson's assistance and expertise with this aspect of the translation is gratefully acknowledged.

Technical disease terms that require an explanation are marked by consistent capitalization in the running translation text. Definitions and explanations of these terms can be found in the Glossary. My entries there are based on explanations from early classical literature, most notably the Zhū Bìng Yuán Hòu Lùn that was completed in 610 CE.

Another topic that requires a word of caution is the specific part of plants in particular, but also of some animals, that may be used for medicinal purposes, with the effect described in the text. In some entries, the part is specified in the name (皮 *pí* "bark," 實 *shí* "fruit/seed," 花 huā "flower," etc.), but more often than not, this information is unfortunately missing. In such cases, the English common name only identifies the plant to reflect a literal translation, while the scientific identification provides the additional information on the plant part used, whenever that has been established with reasonable certainty. To avoid the risk of potentially misleading the reader, I have refrained from adding any extra information unless my critical historian's mind, and the academic consensus of Chinese and Western researchers with much more time and resources on their hands, have firmly and unequivocally accepted such additions, as in the case of the entry on *rénshēn* referring to the root.

2. Ruminations on Terminology

For the present book, I have intentionally restrained myself from writing too many sinological footnotes that discuss details of terminological choices of limited or no consequence to a "normal" reader. Here I just want to briefly draw attention to a few characters or phrases that are particularly significant for the present translation.

I have rendered the character 毒 *dú* as "toxin" or "toxic" in the present translation, depending on its grammatical function. Most importantly, it is used in each entry in the phrases 無毒 *wú dú* or 有毒 *yǒu dú*, translated as "toxic" or "non-toxic" respectively. For each substance, the text gives information on the "toxicity" right after the categorization into the Five Flavors (五味 *wǔ wèi*, namely sour, salty, sweet, bitter, and acrid) and Four Qì (四氣 *sì qì*, often translated as "thermodynamic qualities," namely cold, hot, cool, and warm). Given the use of this text as a materia medica, in other words, as a collection of information on substances recommended for human consumption for the purpose of improving or preserving health and longevity, we are led to wonder: Why would a full third of this text be classified as "toxic," namely the so-called "lower" category of medicinals that are associated with earth, identified as "assistants and messengers," and said to "eliminate the evil qì of cold and heat, break up accumulations and gatherings, and cure diseases"? And then there is the middle category of "vassals" who are "in charge of nurturing the Heavenly nature," about whom the text warns: "Some of them are poisonous and some are not, so deliberate their suitability carefully." And why would the substances with the highest efficacy, which are actually able to "treat disease" (治病 *zhì bìng*), be classified as the lowest category, directly contrary to the way in which most modern doctors would rank them?

To cite just one example, the medicinal effect of the substance *qínjiāo*, *Zanthoxylum bungeanum* (Shenxi pepper; page 256), which is classified as toxic, is described in this way: "It treats wind evil qì, warms the center, gets rid of cold-related *Bì* Impediment, makes the teeth firm, grows the hair on the head, and brightens the eyes." These effects certainly make it look like a highly useful substance. More significantly, the text continues: "Consumed over a long period of time, it lightens the body, makes the complexion beautiful, allows you to withstand aging, increases the years, and facilitates the breakthrough of spirit [illumination]." How do we reconcile this description, and the advice on long-term consumption, with its classification as "toxic"?

This entry in fact might shed light not only on the meaning of 毒 *dú* ("toxic/toxin"), but also on two other phrases of great significance for this translation project: The phrases 久服 *jiǔ fú* ("consumed over a long time") and 通神 *tōng shén*, which I have ended up translating with considerable awkwardness as "facilitate the breakthrough of spirit [illumination]."

Let us first return to our consideration of the meaning of toxicity in The Divine Farmer's Classic of Materia Medica. When we look at the categorization of substances as toxic (or the sub-category of slightly toxic) or non-toxic, it becomes clear that our contemporary, scientific or popular, meaning of "toxic" does not fit neatly into the ancient Chinese meaning of *dú* 毒. For example, why are *shíliúhuáng* 石硫黃 (sulfur; page 284) and *máfén* 麻蕡 (hemp seed; page 282) categorized as "toxic" when *dānshā* 丹砂 (cinnabar, a.k.a. mercuric sulfide; page 143) and *fēngzǐ* 蜂子 (wasp; page 175) are said to be "non-toxic"?

For an answer, we need to recall the primary intention and authorship and audience of the information contained in this text. Today, the *Divine Farmer's Classic of Materia Medica* is considered one of the most important classics in Chinese Medicine and is therefore treasured deeply by students and practitioners of this form of medicine. For many centuries, physicians have found insights in this text into the medicinal effect of substances, to support their practice of treating disease and alleviating their patients' suffering. Nevertheless, we must never forget that our modern understanding of the scope and goals of "medicine" or of "materia medica" was very different from the early notions of 醫 *yī* ("medicine") and of 本草 *běncǎo* ("roots and grasses," which I have translated as "materia medica").

As expressed in most classical medical literature in one form or another, the creators of the early Chinese classics, for example, idealized the approach of "treating disease before it arises" (治未病 *zhì wéi bìng*). Even more drastically, many if not most of the leading researchers of natural science in early and medieval China were actively engaged in efforts to physically and spiritually transform their natural body and transcend the limitations of its mortal human form (形 *xíng*), to avoid or transform death and turn into spirit immortals (仙 *xiān*). We must never forget this alchemical background, which differs so greatly from our own intentions for the use of "medicinal" substances.

From this perspective, the term 毒 *dú* "toxin/toxic" takes on a different meaning. Looked at from the perspective of etymology, it is a combination of the two characters 生 *shēng* ("life"), or 草 *cǎo* ("grass") over 毋 *wú* ("do not!"), aptly paraphrased by the famous Swedish linguist Bernhard Karlgren as "forbidden herbs." Early variations of the character include the characters 刀 *dāo* ("knife") or 虫 *chóng* ("insect"), both things that are associated with harming people. So in other contexts, the character can safely be equated with the English term "toxin," which is why I have chosen to do so here as well. The issue, in other words, is not that the Chinese character 毒 means something different from the English word "toxin," but that it carries a specific meaning here that we must keep in mind. I used to explain it as "medicinal efficacy" in the context of this book, but such an explanation only works if we are clear on the different meaning of "medicinal" in the early texts: Yes, treating disease was one desired outcome of using natural substances, but the actual transformation of the physical body, which in cases like the long-term consumption of cinnabar and other minerals might involve inflicting real and permanent harm on it, was a higher and more important goal, associated with the connection to heaven.

The long-term consumption of substances aimed at the gradual alchemical transformation of the body is therefore an essential aspect of the information presented in The *Divine Farmer's Classic of Materia Medica*. The reader can gain a better understanding of the specific goals of this alchemical transformation by looking at the effects of substances described after the phrase 久服 *jiǔ fú* ("Consumed over a long time"). The most important effects are related to three actions: lightening the body (輕身 *qīng shēn*), staving off aging (or extending the years or some variation thereof, 耐老延年 *nài lǎo yán niān*), and, the most difficult phrase to translate in the entire book, "facilitate the breakthrough of spirit [illumination] (通神 *tōng shén*). The goal of preventing or reversing aging requires no more explanation here. Similarly, "lightening the body" is an effect that the reader can experience on a personal level. In my mind, I read it literally, in the sense that the body feels light and airy, instead of being weighted down in such a way that it requires effort to keep it upright or move limbs.

Resolving the conundrum of translating the expression 通神 *tōng shén*, or its common relative 通神明 *tōng shénmíng*, proves much harder. I have changed my translation dozens of times, from the awfully prosaic "unclog the spirit" to the unclear "connect [the body's?] spirit(s) with [Heaven's brightness]," to the poetic but maybe too free "induce a state of lucid connectedness," to its current version, "facilitate the breakthrough of spirit [illumination]." There are almost as many possibilities for interpreting and translating this phrase as there are readers and translators. I look forward to receiving your comments but do not anticipate a solution that will satisfy many discerning readers. I would in fact have much preferred to leave it in *pīnyīn* but have decided against this practice, to keep the text accessible to readers with no background in Chinese.

Neither 通 *tōng* nor 神 *shén* are characters that are easily translated into any modern language. In the case of 神 *shén*, the English "spirit" or "Spirit" may express the connection to Heavenly Spirit, or to spirit in the sense of a person's vitality or esprit, but it leaves out the plurality of "spirits" that inhabit the human body, surround it in the natural environment, and connect it upwards with Heaven. Those of you who practice Chinese medicine or any of the Chinese arts of self-cultivation know that *shén* is just *shén*, and that "spirit," whether in the singular or plural, is indeed a questionable and uneasy English rendition of one of the most important concepts in Chinese culture. Etymologically, you could perhaps explain it as the act of "stretching upward toward something sacred," a place or entity that most people associate with the Chinese concept of "Heaven."

Concerning the character 通 *tōng*, it implies the idea of connecting, of penetrating through all the way to the end, of unclogging, as in the medical action of 通經 *tōng jīng*, of unclogging the channels (or the menstrual period) by removing obstructions, of restoring free flow. Again, this is perhaps a concept that is more easily grasped by experiencing the effect of this action on the human body in person. In the oldest Chinese dictionary *Shuō Wén Jiě Zì* 說文解字, the character 通 is defined as 達 *dá*, "to reach." In addition, the classical meanings of the character include notions like to pervade, to comprehend, to move forcefully, and to communicate and interact. In my mind, especially in the phrase 通神明 *tōng shénmíng* ("facilitate the breakthrough of spirit illumination"), the medicinal substance that is said to have this effect allows the light of the spirit or spirits to shine through, to illuminate the farthest reaches of "Under Heaven" like the supercharged beam of a magical flashlight. But ultimately, this phrase may just be impossible to express in a modern Western language but can only be grasped on a non-rational level, because it is beyond the limitations of our linguistic capacities.

In conclusion, I hope that you enjoy pondering these sorts of conundrums as much as I do and that this book invites you to ponder a few new ones.

> "Be patient toward all that is unsolved in your heart and try to love the questions themselves… Do not now seek the answers, which cannot be given you because you would not be able to live them. And the point is, to live everything. Live the questions now. Perhaps you will then gradually, without noticing it, live along some distant day into the answer."
>
> Rainer Maria Rilke, *Letters to a Young Poet*

序錄

PREFACE

（一）上藥一百二十種為君，主養命以應天，無毒，多服久服不傷人，欲輕身益氣不老延年者，本《上經》。

（二）中藥一百二十種為臣，主養性以應人，無毒，有毒，斟酌其宜，欲遏病補虛羸者，本《中經》。

Section One

(1) The upper-level medicinals consist of 120 types. These function as rulers. They are in charge of nurturing Destiny and thereby correspond to Heaven. They are non-toxic and, [even] when taken in large quantities or over a long time, do not harm the person. If you want to lighten the body, boost qì, avoid aging, and extend your lifespan, root [your prescriptions] in the upper [section of the] Classic.[1]

(2) The mid-level medicinals consist of 120 types. These function as vassals. They are in charge of nurturing the Heavenly Nature and thereby correspond to Humanity. Some of them are toxic and some are not, so deliberate their suitability carefully. If you want to check illness and supplement vacuity emaciation, root [your prescriptions] in the middle [section of the] Classic.

---

1 "Upper Classic" here clearly refers to the section in the *Divine Farmer's Classic of Materia Medica* that covers the upper-level medicinals.

（三）下藥一百二十五種為佐使，主治病以應地，多毒，不可久服，欲除寒熱邪氣、破積聚、愈疾者，本《下經》。

（四）三品合三百六十五種，法三百六十五度。一度應一日，以應一歲。

(3) The lower-level medicinals consist of 125 types. These function as the assistants and messengers. They are in charge of treating illness and thereby correspond to Earth. In most cases, they are toxic and may not be taken over a long period of time. If you want to eliminate the evil qì of cold and heat, break up accumulations and gatherings, and cure diseases, root [your prescriptions] in the lower [section of the Classic].

(4) The three levels combine to a total of 365 types, precedented by the 365 measures. One measure corresponds to one day, and [the whole Classic] thereby corresponds to one year.

（一）藥有君、臣、佐、使，以相宣攝。合和者，宜用一君、二臣、五佐。又可一君、三臣、九佐、使也。

（二）藥有陰陽配合，子、母、兄、弟，根、莖、花、實、草、石、骨、肉。

（三）有單行者，有相須者，有使者，有相畏者，有相惡者，有相反者，有相殺者。

Section Two

(1) Among the medicinals, there are rulers, vassals, assistants, and messengers. By means of [these roles], they can have a disseminating or containing effect on each other. To combine them harmoniously, you should use one ruler, two vassals, and five assistants. It is also possible to use one ruler, three vassals, and nine assistants and messengers.

(2) Among the medicinals, there are matching pairs of yīn and yáng, there are child and mother and older sibling and younger sibling [relationships]; and there are roots, stalks, flowers, fruits, herbs, stones, bones, and flesh.

(3) There are those who act on their own, those who need each other, those who serve as messengers for each other, those who fear each other, those who are averse to each other, those who counteract each other, and those who kill each other.

（四）凡此七情，和合時視之，當用相須、相使者良，勿用相惡、相反者。

（五）若有毒宜制，可用相畏、相殺者。不爾，勿合用也。

(4) In all cases, you must observe these seven mutual relationships when combining medicinals. It is excellent to use those that need each other or serve as messengers for each other. Do not use ones that are averse to each other or counteract each other.

(5) If they are toxic, it is appropriate to trim down [this effect]. [For this purpose,] you can use [medicinals] that fear or kill each other. Otherwise, do not use them in combination!

（一）藥有酸、鹹、甘、苦、辛五味，又有寒、熱、溫、涼四氣，及有毒、無毒，陰乾、暴乾，采治時月，生熟，土地所出，真、偽、陳、新，並各有法。

（二）藥有宜丸者，宜散者，宜水煮者，宜酒浸者，宜膏煎者，亦有一物兼宜者，亦有不可入湯酒者，並隨藥性，不得違越。

Section Three

(1) Medicinals have the Five Flavors of sour, salty, sweet, bitter, and acrid, as well as the Four Qì of cold, hot, warm, and cool. In addition, there are those that are toxic and those that are not. Whether they are dried in the shade or in the sun, the time and month when they are gathered and prepared, whether they are used raw or cooked, the locale where they come from, and whether they are genuine or false, and old or fresh, these [aspects] also each have their precedents.

(2) Among the medicinals, some should be [prepared] as pills, some as powders, some should be decocted in water, some steeped in liquor, some simmered in grease. There are also some substances that can be prepared in a number of ways and those that must not be added to water or liquor. For all of these you must follow the inherent nature of the medicinal and may not go against it.

（一）凡欲治病，先察其源，候其病機。

（二）五臟未虛，六腑未竭，血脈未亂，精神未散，服藥必活。

（三）若病已成，可得半愈。

（四）病勢已過，命將難全。

Section Four

(1) Whenever you want to treat illness, first examine its source and observe the pathomechanism.

(2) When the five *zàng* organs are not vacuous yet, the six *fǔ* organs are not critically depleted yet, the flow of the blood in the vessels is not disordered yet, and the essence spirit is not yet scattered, taking medicinals invariably results in survival.

(3) If the illness has already matured, you can obtain a cure in half of all cases.

(4) If the force of the illness has already become too great, [the patient's] allotted lifespan will be difficult to complete.

(一) 若用毒治病,先起如黍粟,病去及止,不去倍之,不去十之,取去為度。

(二) 治寒以熱藥,治熱以寒藥。

(三) 飲食不消,以吐下藥。鬼疾、蠱毒,以毒藥。癰腫瘡瘤,以瘡藥。風濕,以風濕藥。

(四) 各隨其所宜。

Section Five

(1) If you use toxic [medicinals] to treat illness, first begin with an amount the size of a millet grain. If you get rid of the illness, stop. If you do not get rid of it, double [the amount]. If you [still] do not get rid of it, increase it tenfold. Use getting rid of the illness as your measure.

(2) To treat cold, use hot medicinals. To treat heat, use cold medicinals.

(3) For inability to eliminate food and drink, use medicinals that induce vomiting or downward movement. For being struck by ghosts or by *Gǔ* Toxin, use toxic medicinals. For welling-abscesses, external sores, and tumors, use medicinals for treating external sores. For wind and dampness, use wind- and dampness-treating medicinals.

(4) Use each in accordance with what it is appropriate for.

（一）病在胸膈以上者，先食後服藥。

（二）病在心腹以下者，先服藥而後食。

（三）病在四肢血脈者，宜空腹而在旦。

（四）病在骨髓者，宜飽滿而在夜。

Section Six

(1) If the illness is located above the chest and diaphragm, eat first and take the medicine afterwards.

(2) If the illness is below the heart and abdomen, first take the medicine and then eat afterwards.

(3) If the illness is in the four limbs and the blood vessels, take the medicine at dawn on an empty stomach.

(4) If the illness is in the bones and marrow, take the medicine at night after you have stuffed yourself.

（一）夫大病之主，有中風、傷寒、溫瘧、中惡、霍亂、大腹、水腫、腸澼、下利、大小便不通、奔豚上氣、咳逆、嘔吐、黃疸、消渴、留飲、癖食、堅積、癥瘕、驚邪、癲癇、鬼注、喉痹、齒痛、耳聾、目盲、金瘡、踒折、癰腫、惡瘡、痔瘻、瘻瘤、男子五勞七傷、虛乏羸瘦，女子帶下、崩中、血閉，陰瘡、蟲蛇、蠱毒所傷。

（二）此皆大略宗兆。其間變動枝葉，各宜依端緒以取之。

Section Seven

(1) Now, the major [categories of] illness are wind strike, cold damage, warm malaria, malignity strike, cholera, enlarged abdomen and water swelling, dysentery and diarrhea, stopped urination and defecation, Bolting Piglet qì ascent, cough and counterflow, retching and vomiting, jaundice, dispersion thirst, lodged rheum, food aggregations, hardness and gatherings, concretions and conglomerations, fright evil, Epilepsy, ghost influx, throat *Bì* Impediment, toothache, deafness, blindness, incised wounds, sprains and breaks, welling-abscesses, malign sores, Hemorrhoids and fistulas, goiters; in men the Five Taxations and Seven Damages, vacuity fatigue, and emaciation; in women vaginal discharge, vaginal hemorrhaging, and blood blockage; and injuries from genital sores, insect and snake bites, and *gǔ* poisoning.

(2) This is all just a rough outline, based on exemplary signs. Between these [major illness categories], there will be changes and movement in the branches and leaves. In each case, rely on the fine threads of evidence to thereby gain [an understanding of the illness].

上藥

Upper Medicinals

草部

Herbs

菖蒲

一名昌陽
味辛，溫，無毒

治風寒濕痹，欬逆上氣，開心孔，補五臟，通九竅，明耳目，出音聲。久服輕身，不忘，不迷惑，延年。生池澤。

---

chāngpú

rhizome of *Acorus gramineus* (sweet flag)
ALTERNATE NAME: *chāngyáng* "splendid yáng"
acrid flavor, warm, non-toxic

Treats wind-, cold-, and damp-related *Bì* Impediment, and counterflow cough with ascent of qì; opens up the apertures of the heart; supplements the five *zàng* organs; unclogs the Nine Orifices; brightens the ears and eyes; and makes the sound of the voice come forth. Consumed over a long time, it lightens the body, staves off forgetfulness and confusion, and extends the years. Grows in ponds and marshes.

菊花

一名節華
味苦,平,無毒

治風頭, 頭眩腫痛,目欲脫,淚出,皮膚死肌,惡風,濕痹。久服利血氣,輕身,耐老,延年。生川澤及田野。

---

júhuā

flower of *Chrysanthemum x morifolium* (chrysanthemum)
ALTERNATE NAME: *jiéhuá* "node flower"
bitter flavor, balanced, non-toxic

Treats wind-head; dizziness, swelling, and pain in the head; eyes about to protrude and tearing; dead flesh in the skin; aversion to wind; and damp-related *Bì* Impediment. Consumed over a long time, it disinhibits blood and qì, lightens the body, allows you to withstand aging, and extends the years. Grows in rivers and marshes, as well as in open fields.

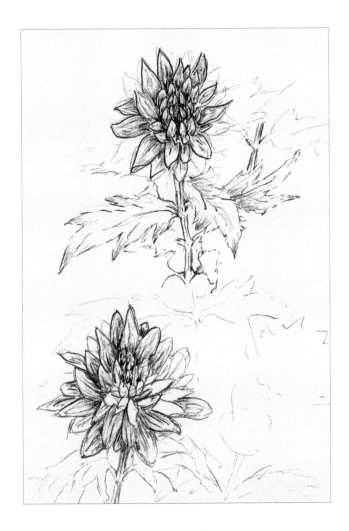

Sketch 1 - *júhuā*

人參

一名人銜,一名鬼蓋
味甘,微寒,無毒

主補五臟,安精神,定魂魄,止驚悸,除邪氣,明目,開心益智。久服輕身,延年。生山谷。

---

rénshēn

root of *Panax ginseng* (ginseng)
ALTERNATE NAMES: *rénxián* "human snaffle,"
guǐgài "ghost cover"
sweet flavor, slightly cold, non-toxic

Indicated for supplementing the five *zàng* organs, calming the essence spirit(s) and settling the *hún* and *pò* souls, stopping fright palpitations, expelling evil qì, brightening the eyes, and opening up the heart and boosting wisdom. Consumed over a long time, it lightens the body and extends the years. Grows in mountain valleys.

天門冬

一名顛勒
味苦,平,無毒

治諸暴風濕偏痹,強骨髓,殺三蟲,去伏屍。久服輕身,益氣,延年。生山谷。

---

tiānméndōng

"heaven gate winter"
tuber of *Asparagus cochinchinensis* (Chinese asparagus)
ALTERNATE NAME: *diānlè* "apex fastener"
bitter flavor, balanced, non-toxic

Treats all sorts of sudden wind- and damp-related unilateral *Bì* Impediment, strengthens the bones and marrow, kills the Three Worms, and gets rid of Lurking Corpse [syndrome]. Consumed over a long time, it lightens the body, boosts qì, and extends the years. Grows in mountain valleys.

甘草

一名美草，一名蜜甘
味甘，平，無毒

治五臟六腑寒熱邪氣，堅筋骨，長肌肉，倍力，金瘡，尰，解毒。久服輕身，延年。生川谷。

---

gāncǎo

"sweet herb"

root of *Glycyrrhiza uralensis* (licorice)

ALTERNATE NAMES: *měicǎo* "delicious herb,"
mìgān "honey sweet"

sweet flavor, balanced, non-toxic

Treats evil qì of cold and heat in the five *zàng* and six *fǔ* organs, makes the sinews and bones firm, grows the flesh and multiplies strength, [treats] incised wounds and swellings in the legs, and resolves toxin. Consumed over a long time, it lightens the body and extends the years. Grows in river valleys.

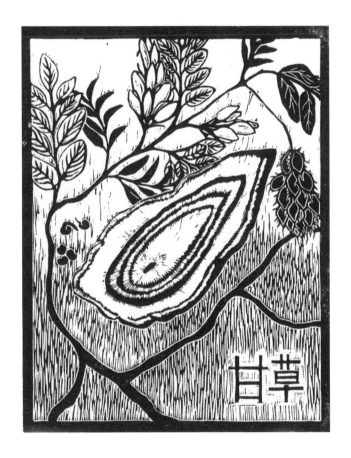

Block Print 1 - *gāncǎo*

乾地黃

一名地髓
味甘,寒,無毒

治折跌絕筋、傷中,逐血痹,填骨髓,長肌肉。作湯,除寒熱、積聚,除痹。生者尤良。久服輕身,不老。生川澤。

---

gāndìhuáng

"dried earth yellow"
dried root of *Rehmannia glutinosa* (rehmannia)
ALTERNATE NAME: *dìsuǐ* "marrow of the earth"
sweet flavor, cold, non-toxic

Treats fractures, falls, severed sinews, and damage to the center; drives out blood *Bì* Impediment; fills in the bones and marrow; and grows flesh. Prepared as a decoction, it gets rid of cold and heat, accumulations and gatherings, and *Bì* Impediment. Used fresh, it is particularly excellent. Consumed over a long time, it lightens the body and staves off aging. Grows in rivers and marshes.

朮

一名山薊
味苦,溫,無毒

治風寒濕痺、死肌、痙、疸。止汗,除熱,消食。作煎餌。久服輕身,延年,不飢。生山谷。

---

zhú

rhizome of *Atractylodes macrocephala* (atractylodes)
ALTERNATE NAME: *shānjì*, "mountain thistle"
bitter flavor, warm, non-toxic

Treats wind-, cold-, and damp-related *Bì* Impediment, dead flesh, tetany, and jaundice; stops sweating; gets rid of heat; and disperses food. Prepare as fried cakes. Consumed over a long time, it lightens the body, extends the years, and staves off hunger. Grows in mountain valleys.

菟絲子

一名菟蘆
味辛,平,無毒

主續絕傷,補不足,益氣力,肥健。汁,去面䵟。久服明目,輕身,延年。生川澤野,蔓延草木之上。

---

tùsīzǐ

seed of *Cuscuta chinensis* (dodder seed)
ALTERNATE NAME: *tùlú* "*tù* reed"
acrid flavor, balanced, non-toxic

Indicated for reconnecting damage from severance, supplementing insufficiencies, boosting qì and strength, and making you plump and healthy. The juice gets rid of black spots in the face. Consumed over a long time, it brightens the eyes, lightens the body, and extends the years. Grows in rivers and marshes and in open fields, forms vines that climb on top of herbs and trees.

牛膝

一名百倍
味苦,平,無毒

治寒濕痿痺、四肢拘攣、膝痛不可屈伸,逐血氣,傷熱,火爛,墮胎。久服輕身,耐老。生川谷。

---

niúxī

"cow's knee"
root of *Achyranthes bidentata* (achyranthes)
ALTERNATE NAME: *bǎibèi* "hundredfold"
bitter flavor, balanced, non-toxic

Treats wind- and damp-related wilting and *Bì* Impediment, hypertonicity of the four limbs, and pain and inability to bend or stretch in the knees; drives out [pathological] blood and qì; [and treats] heat damage, putrefaction due to fire, and miscarriage. Consumed over a long time, it lightens the body and allows you to withstand aging. Grows in river valleys.

茺蔚子

一名益母,一名益明,一名大札
味辛,微溫,無毒

主明目,益精,除水氣。久服輕身。莖,治癮疹癢,可作浴湯。生海濱、池澤。

---

chōngwèizǐ

seed of *Leonurus heterophyllus*[1] (Chinese motherwort)
ALTERNATE NAMES: *yìmǔ* "boost the mother,"
yìmíng "boost brightness,"
dàzhá "great bundle of wooden slats"
acrid flavor, slightly warm, non-toxic

Indicated for brightening the eyes, boosting essence, and getting rid of water qì. Consumed over a long time, it lightens the body. The stalks treat dormant papules with itching. They can be prepared as a medicinal bath. Grows on the shores of large bodies of water and in ponds and marshes.

女萎

一名左眄,一名玉竹
味甘,平,無毒

治中風暴熱,不能動搖,胅筋結肉,諸不足。久服去面黑䵟,好顏色,潤澤,輕身,不老。生川谷及丘陵。

---

nǚwěi

stalk of *Clematis apiifolia* (October clematis)
ALTERNATE NAMES: *zuǒmiǎn* "left squinting,"
yùzhú "jade bamboo"
sweet flavor, balanced, non-toxic

Treats wind strike with sudden heat, inability to move and shake, swollen sinews and knotted flesh, and all sorts of insufficiencies. Consumed over a long time, it gets rid of black spots in the face, beautifies the facial complexion, moistens and lubricates, lightens the body, and staves off aging. Grows in river valleys and on hills.

防葵

一名梨蓋
味辛,寒,無毒

治疝瘕,腸泄,膀胱熱結,溺不下,欬逆,溫瘧,癲癇,驚邪,狂走。久服堅骨髓,益氣輕身。生川谷。

---

fángkuí

root of *Peucedanum japonicum* (fangkui peucedanum)
ALTERNATE NAME: *lígài* "pear cover"
acrid flavor, cold, non-toxic

Treats *shàn*-type ("mounding") conglomerations, intestinal diarrhea, heat bind in the bladder, inability to move urine down, cough with counterflow, warm malaria, Epilepsy, fright evil, and manic wandering. Consumed over a long time, it makes the bones and marrow firm, boosts qì, and lightens the body. Grows in river valleys.

柴胡

一名地熏。
味苦,平,無毒。

治心腹,去腸胃中結氣、飲食積聚、寒熱邪氣,推陳致新。久服輕身,明目,益精。生川谷。

---

cháihú

root of *Bupleurum chinense* (hare's ear)
ALTERNATE NAME: *dìxūn* "earth cense"
bitter flavor, balanced, non-toxic

Treats the heart and abdomen; gets rid of bound qì in the intestines and stomach, of accumulations and gatherings of food and drink, and of evil qì of cold and heat; and pushes out the old to usher in the new. Consumed over a long time, it lightens the body, brightens the eyes, and boosts essence. Grows in river valleys.

麥門冬

秦名羊韭，齊名愛韭，楚名馬韭，越名羊韭
味甘，平，無毒

治心腹結氣，傷中，傷飽，胃絡脈絕，羸瘦，短氣。久服輕身，不老，不饑。生川谷及堤阪肥土石間久廢處。

---

màiméndōng

tuber of *Ophiopogon japonicus* (Japanese hyacinth)
ALTERNATE NAMES: in Qín, *yángjiǔ* "sheep leek";
in Qí, *àijiǔ* "love leek"; in Chǔ, *mǎjiǔ* "horse leek";
in Yuè, *yángjiǔ* "sheep leek"
sweet flavor, balanced, non-toxic

Treats bound qì in the heart and abdomen, damage to the center, damage from overeating, severance of the flow in the stomach network vessels, gauntness, and shortness of breath. Consumed over a long time, it lightens the body and staves off aging and hunger. Grows in river valleys as well as in the fertile soil on embankments and hillsides, between rocks, and in long-abandoned locations.

獨活

一名羌活，一名羌青，一名護羌使者
味苦，平，無毒

治風寒所擊，金瘡，止痛，奔豚，癇，痓，女子疝瘕。久服輕身，耐老。生川谷。

---

dúhuó

"singularly enlivening"
root and rhizome of *Angelica pubescens* (pubescent angelica)
ALTERNATE NAMES: *qiānghuó* "life of the Qiāng [tribe],"
qiāngqīng "Qiāng green-blue,"
hùqiāngshǐzhě "emissary who protects the Qiāng [tribe]"
bitter flavor, balanced, non-toxic

Treats attacks by wind and cold, and incised wounds; stops pain; and [treats] Bolting Piglet (*bēn tún*), Seizures, tetany, and women's *shàn*-type ("mounding") conglomerations. Consumed over a long time, it lightens the body and allows you to withstand aging. Grows in river valleys.

車前子

一名當道
味甘,寒,無毒

治氣癃,止痛,利水道小便,除濕痺。久服輕身,耐老。生平澤、丘陵、阪道中。

---

chēqiánzǐ

"in front of the cart seed"
seed of *Plantago asiatica* (plantain seed)
ALTERNATE NAME: *dāngdào* "right in the path"
sweet flavor, cold, non-toxic

Treats qì dribbling urinary block, stops pain, disinhibits the waterways and urine, and gets rid of damp-related *Bì* Impediment. Consumed over a long time, it lightens the body and allows you to withstand aging. Grows in marshy flatlands, on hills, and in the middle of hillside trails.

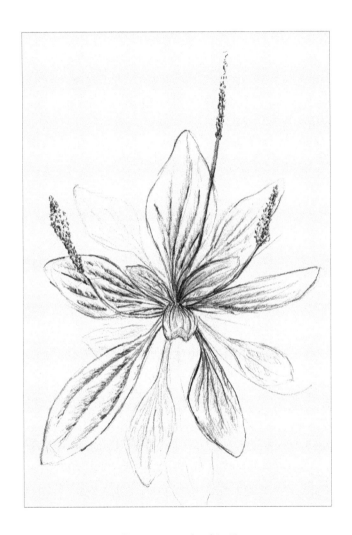

Sketch 2 - *chēqiánzǐ*

木香

一名木蜜
味辛,溫,無毒

治邪氣,辟毒、疫、溫、鬼,強志,治淋露。久服不夢寤魘寐。生山谷。

---

mùxiāng

"wood fragrance"
root of *Aucklandia lappa* (costusroot)
ALTERNATE NAME: *mùmì* "wood honey"
acrid flavor, warm, non-toxic

Treats evil qì; wards off toxins, epidemics, [pathogenic] warmth, and demons; strengthens the will; and treats being drenched by rain and dew. Consumed over a long time, it staves off being awakened from your dreams by nightmares. Grows in mountain valleys.

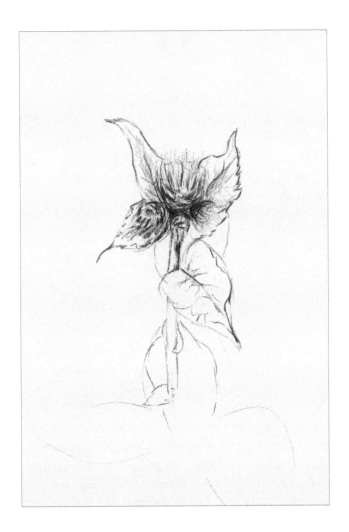

Sketch 3 - *mùxiāng*

薯蕷

一名山芋，秦、楚名玉延，郑、
越名土薯，齊、趙名山羊
味甘，溫，無毒

治傷中，補虛羸，除寒熱邪氣，補中，益氣力，長肌肉。久服耳目聰明，輕身，不饑，延年。生山谷。

---

shǔyù

root of *Dioscorea opposita* (potato yam)
ALTERNATE NAMES: *shānyù* "mountain taro"; in Qín and Chǔ, *yùyán* "jade extension"; in Zhèng and Yuè, *tǔzhū* "local yam"; in Qí and Zhào, *shānyáng* "mountain goat"
sweet flavor, warm, non-toxic

Treats damage to the center, emptiness and gauntness, gets rid of the evil qì of cold and heat, supplements the center, boosts qì and strength, and makes the flesh grow. Consumed over a long time, it makes the ears and eyes sharp and bright, lightens the body, staves off hunger, and extends the years. Grows in mountain valleys.

薏苡仁

一名解蠡
味甘,微寒,無毒

治筋急拘攣、不可屈伸、風濕痹,下氣。久服輕身,益氣。其根,下三蟲。生平澤及田野。

---

yìyǐrén

seed kernel of *Coix lachrymae-jobi* (Job's tears)
ALTERNATE NAME: *jiělí* "split calabash"
sweet flavor, slightly cold, non-toxic

Treats hypertonicity of the sinews, inability to bend or stretch, and wind- and damp-related *Bì* Impediment; and moves qì down. Consumed over a long time, it lightens the body and boosts qì. Its root moves the Three Worms down and out. Grows in marshy flatlands and open fields.

澤瀉

一名水瀉，一名芒芋，一名鵠瀉
味甘，寒，無毒

治風寒濕痹、乳難，消水，養五臟，益氣力，肥健。久服耳目聰明，不饑，延年，輕身，面生光，能行水上。生池澤。

---

zéxiè

"marsh drainer"
rhizome of *Alisma plantago-aquatica* (water plantain)
ALTERNATE NAMES: *shuǐxiè* "water drainer,"
mángyù "máng taro," *húxiè* "swan drainer"
sweet flavor, cold, non-toxic

Treats wind-, cold-, and damp-related *Bì* Impediment and problems with breastfeeding; disperses water; nurtures the five *zàng* organs; boosts qì and strength; and makes you plump and healthy. Consumed over a long time, it makes the ears and eyes sharp and bright, staves off hunger, extends the years, lightens the body, makes the face glow, and gives the ability to walk on water. Grows in ponds and marshes.

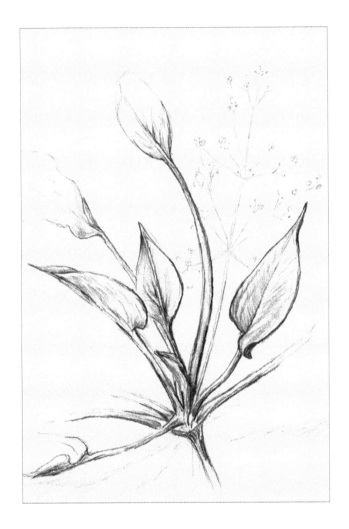

Sketch 4 - *zéxiè*

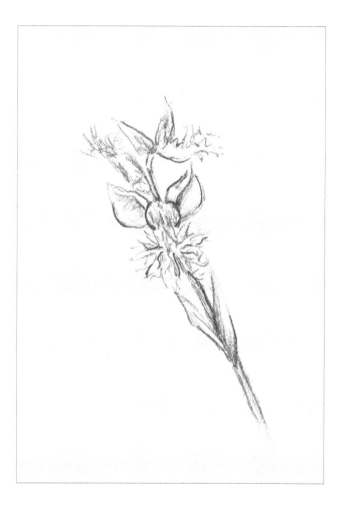

Sketch 5 - *yuǎnzhì*

遠志

一名棘菀,一名葽繞,一名細草
味苦,溫,無毒

治欬逆、傷中,補不足,除邪氣,利九竅,益智慧,耳目聰明,不忘,強志,倍力。久服輕身,不老。葉名小草。生川谷。

---

yuǎnzhì

"making the will far-reaching"
root of *Polygala tenuifolia*[2] (milkwort)
ALTERNATE NAMES: *jíwǎn* "thistle aster,"
yāorào, *xìcǎo* "tiny herb"
bitter flavor, warm, non-toxic

Treats counterflow cough and damage to the center; supplements insufficiency; gets rid of evil qì; disinhibits the Nine Orifices; boosts wisdom; makes the ears and eyes sharp and bright; staves off forgetfulness; strengthens the will; and multiplies strength. Consumed over a long time, it lightens the body and staves off aging. The leaves are called *xiǎocǎo* "small herb." Grows in river valleys.

龍膽

一名陵游
味苦,寒,無毒

治骨間寒熱、驚癇、邪氣,續絕傷,定五臟,殺蠱毒。久服益智,不忘,輕身,耐老。生山谷。

---

lóngdǎn

"dragon's gall"
root and rhizome of *Gentiana scabra* (gentian)
ALTERNATE NAME: *língyóu* "mound drifter"
bitter flavor, cold, non-toxic

Treats cold and heat in the space of the bones, fright Seizures, and evil qì; reconnects damage from severance; settles the five *zàng* organs; and kills *Gǔ* Toxin. Consumed over a long time, it boosts wisdom, staves off forgetfulness, lightens the body, and allows you to withstand aging. Grows in mountain valleys.

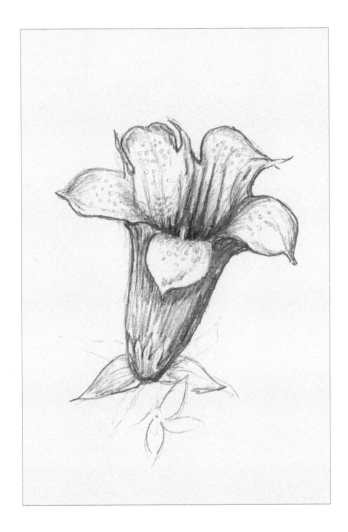

Sketch 6 - *lóngdǎn*

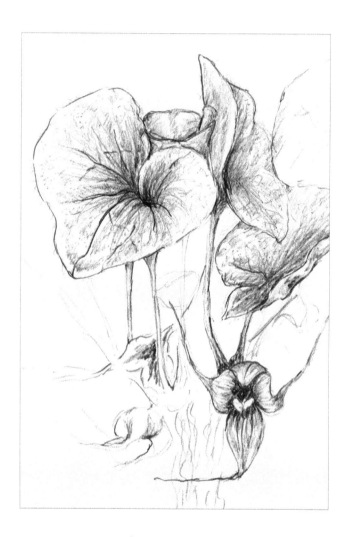

Sketch 7 - *xìxīn*

細辛

一名小辛
味辛，溫，無毒

治欬逆，頭痛，百節拘攣，風濕痺痛，死肌。久服明目，利九竅，輕身，長年。生山谷。

---

xìxīn

"fine acridity"
whole plant of *Asarum heteropoides* (asarum)
ALTERNATE NAME: *xiǎoxīn* "small acridity"
acrid flavor, warm, non-toxic

Treats cough with counterflow, headache, hypertonicity in the hundred joints, wind- and damp-related *Bì* Impediment pain, and dead flesh. Consumed over a long time, it brightens the eyes, disinhibits the Nine Orifices, lightens the body, and lengthens the years. Grows in mountain valleys.

石斛

一名林蘭
味甘,平,無毒

治傷中,除痺,下氣,補五臟虛勞、羸瘦,強陰。久服厚腸胃,輕身,延年。生山谷、水傍石上。

---

shíhú

"rock goblet"
whole plant of *Dendrobium nobile* (dendrobium)
ALTERNATE NAME: *línlán* "forest orchid"
sweet flavor, balanced, non-toxic

Treats damage to the center, gets rid of *Bì* Impediment, moves qì down, supplements emptiness and taxation in the five *zàng* organs and gauntness, and strengthens yīn. Consumed over a long time, it plumps out the stomach and intestines, lightens the body, and extends the years. Grows in mountain valleys and on rocks by water.

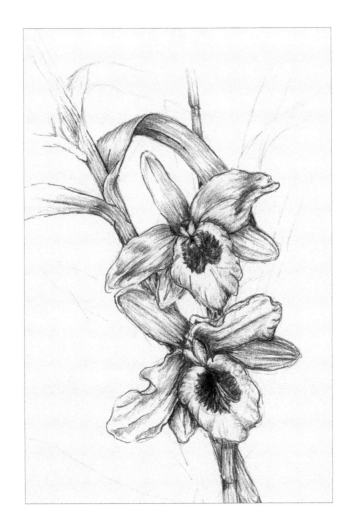

SKETCH 8 - *shíhú*

巴戟天

味辛,微溫,無毒

治大風邪氣、陰痿不起,強筋骨,安五臟,補中,增志,益氣。生山谷。

---

bājǐtiān

root of *Morinda officinalis* (morinda)
acrid flavor, slightly warm, non-toxic

Treats the evil qì of great wind and Yīn Wilt with inability to raise [the penis], strengthens the sinews and bones, calms the five *zàng* organs, supplements the center, increases the will, and boosts qì. Grows in mountain valleys.

白英

一名谷菜
味甘,寒,無毒

治寒熱、八疽、消渴,補中益氣。久服輕身,延年。生山谷。

---

báiyīng

"white bloom"
whole plant of *Solanum lyratum* (climbing nightshade)
ALTERNATE NAME: *gǔcài* ("valley greens")
sweet flavor, cold, non-toxic

Treats cold and heat, the eight [kinds of] flat-abscesses, and dispersion-thirst; and supplements the center and boosts qì. Consumed over a long time, it lightens the body and extends the years. Grows in mountain valleys.

白蒿

味甘,平,無毒

治五臟邪氣、風寒濕痹,補中益氣,長毛髮、令黑,治心懸、少食常饑。久服輕身,耳目聰明,不老。生川澤。

báihāo

whole plant of *Artemisia sieversiana* (Sievers artemisia)
sweet flavor, balanced, non-toxic

Treats evil qì in the five *zàng* organs and wind-, cold-, and damp-related *Bì* Impediment; supplements the center and boosts qì; makes the hair grow long and turns it black; and treats heart suspension and reduced eating and constant hunger. Consumed over a long time, it lightens the body, makes the ears and eyes sharp and bright, and staves off aging. Grows in rivers and marshes.

赤箭

一名離母,一名鬼督郵
味辛,溫,無毒

主殺鬼精物,蠱毒,惡氣。久服益氣力,長陰,肥健,輕身,增年。生川谷。

---

chìjiàn

"red arrow"
rhizome of *Gastrodia elata* (gastrodia)
ALTERNATE NAMES: *límǔ* "detached from the mother,"
guǐdūyóu "ghost inspector"
acrid flavor, warm, non-toxic

Indicated for killing demons and spectral entities, *Gǔ* Toxin, and malign qì. Consumed over a long time, it boosts qì and strength, lengthens yīn,[3] makes you plump and healthy, lightens the body, and increases the years [of life]. Grows in river valleys.

菴閭子

味苦,微寒,無毒。

治五臟瘀血,腹中水氣,臚脹,留熱,風寒濕痺,身體諸痛。久服輕身,延年,不老。生川谷及道邊。

ānlǘzǐ

fruit of *Artemisia keiskeana* (Keiske artemisia seed)
bitter flavor, slightly cold, non-toxic

Treats static blood in the five *zàng* organs; water qì inside the abdomen; distention in the anterior part of the abdomen; lingering heat; wind-, cold-, and damp-related *Bì* Impediment; and all sorts of pains in the body. Consumed over a long time, it lightens the body, extends the years, and staves off aging. Grows in river valleys and on the side of roads.

菥蓂子

一名蔑菥，一名大蕺，一名馬辛
味辛，微溫，無毒

主明目、目痛、淚出，除痹，補五臟，益精光。久服輕身，不老。生川澤及道旁。

---

xīmíngzǐ

seed of *Thlaspi arvense* (pennycress seed)
ALTERNATE NAMES: *mièxī*, *dàjí* "great houttuynia,"
mǎxīn "horse acridity"
acrid flavor, slightly warm, non-toxic

Indicated for brightening the eyes and for eye pain and tearing; getting rid of *Bì* Impediment; supplementing the five *zàng* organs; and boosting the essence brightness.[4] Consumed over a long time, it lightens the body and staves off aging. Grows in rivers and marshes and alongside roads.

蓍實

味苦,平,無毒

主益氣,充肌膚,明目,聰慧先知。久服不饑,不老,輕身。生山谷。

---

shīshí

fruit of *Achillea alpina* (alpine yarrow fruit)
bitter flavor, balanced, non-toxic

Indicated for boosting qì, filling out the skin and flesh, brightening the eyes, and sharpening intelligence and foreknowledge. Consumed over a long time, it staves off hunger and aging and lightens the body. Grows in mountain valleys.

赤芝

一名丹芝
味苦,平,無毒

治胸中結,益心氣,補中,增智慧,不忘。
久食輕身,不老,延年,神仙。生山谷。

---

chìzhī

red conk[5]
fruiting body of red *Ganoderma*
ALTERNATE NAME: *dānzhī* "cinnabar conk"
bitter flavor, balanced, non-toxic

Treats binding inside the chest, boosts heart qì, supplements the center, increases wisdom, and staves off forgetfulness. Eaten over a long time, it lightens the body, staves off aging, extends the years, and [makes you] a spirit immortal. Grows in mountain valleys.

黑芝

一名玄芝
味鹹,平,無毒

治癃,利水道,益腎氣,通九竅,聰察。
久食輕身,不老,延年,神仙。生山谷。

---

hēizhī

black conk
fruiting body of black *Ganoderma*
ALTERNATE NAME: *xuánzhī* "dark conk"
salty flavor, balanced, non-toxic

Treats dribbling urinary block, disinhibits the waterways, boosts kidney qì, unclogs the Nine Orifices, and sharpening perspicacity. Eaten over a long time, it lightens the body, staves off aging, extends the years, and [makes you] a spirit immortal. Grows in mountain valleys.

青芝

一名龍芝
味酸,平,無毒

主明目,補肝氣,安精魂,仁恕。久食輕身,不老,延年,神仙。生山谷。

---

qīngzhī

green-blue conk
fruiting body of green-blue *Ganoderma*
ALTERNATE NAME: *lóngzhī* "dragon conk"
sour flavor, balanced, non-toxic

Indicated for brightening the eyes, supplementing liver qì, putting the essence and calms the *hún* souls, and [producing] compassion. Eaten over a long time, it lightens the body, staves off aging, extends the years, and [makes you] a spirit immortal. Grows in mountain valleys.

白芝

一名玉芝
味辛,平,無毒

治欬逆上氣,益肺氣,通利口鼻,強志意,勇悍,安魄。久食輕身,不老,延年,神仙。生山谷。

---

báizhī

white conk
fruiting body of white *Ganoderma*
ALTERNATE NAME: *yùzhī* "jade conk"
acrid flavor, balanced, non-toxic

Treats counterflow cough with ascent of qì, boosts lung qì, unclogs the mouth and nose, strengthens the will and intention, [produces] valiant courage, and calms the *pò* souls. Eaten over a long time, it lightens the body, staves off aging, extends the years, and [makes you] a spirit immortal. Grows in mountain valleys.

黃芝

一名金芝
味甘,平,無毒

治心腹五邪,益脾氣,安神,忠信和樂。
久食輕身,不老,延年,神仙。生山谷。

---

huángzhī

yellow conk
fruiting body of yellow *Ganoderma*
ALTERNATE NAME: *jīnzhī* "gold conk"
sweet flavor, balanced, non-toxic

Treats the five evils in the heart and abdomen, boosts spleen qì, calms the spirit(s), and [produces] loyalty, sincerity, harmony, and joy. Eaten over a long time, it lightens the body, staves off aging, extends the years, and [makes you] a spirit immortal. Grows in mountain valleys.

紫芝

一名木芝
味甘，溫，無毒

治耳聾，利關節，保神，益精氣，堅筋骨，好顏色。久服輕身，不老，延年。生山谷。

---

zǐzhī

purple conk
fruiting body of purple *Ganoderma*
ALTERNATE NAME: *mùzhī* "wood conk"
sweet flavor, warm, non-toxic

Treats deafness, disinhibits the joints, protects the spirit(s), boosts essence qì, makes the sinews and bones firm, and makes the complexion beautiful. Consumed over a long time, it lightens the body, staves off aging, and extends the years. Grows in mountain valleys.

卷柏

一名萬歲
味辛,溫,無毒

治五臟邪氣,女子陰中寒熱痛,癥瘕,血閉,絕子。久服輕身,和顏色。生山谷石間。

---

juǎnbǎi

whole plant of *Selaginella tamariscina* (spike moss)
ALTERNATE NAME: *wànsuì* "ten-thousand years"
acrid flavor, warm, non-toxic

Treats evil qì in the five *zàng* organs and women's heat and cold pain in the reproductive organs, concretions and conglomerations, blood blockage, and infertility. Consumed over a long time, it lightens the body and harmonizes the complexion. Grows in mountain valleys between rocks.

藍實

味苦,寒,無毒

主解諸毒,殺蠱蚑,疰鬼,螫毒。久服頭不白,輕身。生平澤。

---

lánshí

fruit of *Persicaria tinctoria* (Japanese indigo)
bitter flavor, cold, non-toxic

Indicated for resolving all sorts of toxins, killing *gǔ* poison and spiders, and ghost infixation and poisons from insect bites. Consumed over a long time, it keeps the [hair on the] head from turning white and lightens the body. Grows in marshy flatlands.

蘼蕪

一名薇蕪
味辛,溫,無毒

治欬逆,定驚氣,辟邪惡,除蠱毒、鬼疰,去三蟲。久服通神。生川澤。

---

míwú

foliage and sprout of *Ligusticum wallichii* (Szechuan lovage)
ALTERNATE NAME: *wēiwú* "vetch weed"
acrid flavor, warm, non-toxic

Treats counterflow cough, settles fright qì, wards off evil malignity, expels *gǔ* poison and demonic infixation, and gets rid of the Three Worms. Consumed over a long time, it facilitates the breakthrough of spirit [illumination]. Grows in rivers and marshes.

丹參

一名郤蟬草
味苦，微寒，無毒

治心腹邪氣、腸鳴幽幽如走水、寒熱積聚，破癥，除瘕，止煩滿，益氣。生川谷。

---

dānshēn

"cinnabar *shēn*"
root of *Salvia miltiorrhiza* (sage)
ALTERNATE NAME: *xīchāncǎo* "XĪ cicada herb"
bitter flavor, slightly cold, non-toxic

Treats evil qì in the heart and abdomen, deep rumbling in the intestines as if from running water, and cold- and heat-related accumulations and gatherings; breaks up concretions and gets rid of conglomerations; stops vexation and fullness; and boosts qì. Grows in river valleys.

絡石

一名鯪石
味苦,溫,無毒

治風熱,死肌,癰傷,口乾,舌焦,癰腫不消,喉舌腫,水漿不下。久服輕身,明目,潤澤,好顏色,不老,延年。生川谷。

---

luòshí

"network rock"

vines and foliage of *Trachelospermum jasminoides*

(star jasmine)

ALTERNATE NAME: *língshí* "carp rock"

bitter flavor, warm, non-toxic

Treats wind heat, dead flesh, damage from welling-abscesses, dry mouth, parched tongue, swelling from welling-abscesses that will not disperse, swelling of the throat and tongue, and inability to move water and fluids down. Consumed over a long time, it lightens the body, brightens the eyes, moisturizes and irrigates, beautifies the complexion, staves off aging, and extends the years. Grows in river valleys.

蒺藜子

一名旁通,一名屈人,一名止行,
一名升推,一名豺羽
味苦,溫,無毒

治惡血,破癥結、積聚,喉痺,乳難。久服長肌肉,明目,輕身。生平澤或道傍。

---

jílizǐ

fruit of *Tribulus terrestris* (puncturevine/goathead seed)
ALTERNATE NAMES: *pángtōng* "along-the-side breakthrough,"
qūrén "makes people bend over," *zhǐxíng* "stop moving,"
shēngtuī "rise and push," *cháiyǔ* "jackal feathers"
bitter flavor, warm, non-toxic

Treats malign blood; breaks up concretions, binds, accumulations, and gatherings; [and treats] *Bì* Impediment in the throat and problems with breastfeeding. Consumed over a long time, it makes the flesh grow, brightens the eyes, and lightens the body. Grows in marshy flatlands or along roads.

肉蓯蓉

味甘,微溫,無毒

治五勞七傷,補中,除莖中寒熱痛,養五臟,強陰,益精氣,多子,婦人癥瘕。久服輕身。生山谷。

---

ròucōngróng

fleshy stalk of *Cistanche salsa* or *deserticola* (cistanche)
sweet flavor, slightly warm, non-toxic

Treats the five taxations and Seven Damages, supplements the center, gets rid of cold and heat pain inside the penis, nurtures the five *zàng* organs, strengthens yīn, boosts essence qì, propagates children, and [treats] women's concretions and conglomerations. Consumed over a long time, it lightens the body. Grows in mountain valleys.

防風

一名銅芸
味甘,溫,無毒

治大風,頭眩痛,惡風,風邪,目盲無所見,風行周身,骨節疼痹,煩滿。久服輕身。生川澤。

---

fángfēng

"fend off wind"
root of *Saposhnikovia/Ledebouriella divaricata*[6]
(saposhnikovia/ledebouriella)
ALTERNATE NAME: *tóngyún* "copper rue"
sweet flavor, warm, non-toxic

Treats great wind, dizziness and pain in the head, aversion to wind, wind evil, impaired vision and total loss of eyesight, wind moving all around the body, pain and *Bì* Impediment in the bones and joints, and vexation and fullness. Consumed over a long time, it lightens the body. Grows in rivers and marshes.

蒲黃

味甘,平,無毒

治心腹膀胱寒熱,利小便,止血,消瘀血。久服輕身,益氣力,延年,神仙。生池澤。

---

púhuáng

pollen of *Typha angustata* (cattail pollen)
sweet flavor, balanced, non-toxic

Treats cold and heat in the heart, abdomen, and bladder; disinhibits urine; stops bleeding; and disperses static blood. Consumed over a long time, it lightens the body, boosts qì and strength, extends the years, and [makes you] a spirit immortal. Grows in ponds and marshes.

香蒲

一名睢
味甘，平，無毒

治五臟心下邪氣、口中爛臭，堅齒，明目，聰耳。久服輕身，耐老。生南海池澤。

---

xiāngpú

whole herb of *Typha angustata* (cattail)
ALTERNATE NAME: *suī*
sweet flavor, balanced, non-toxic

Treats evil *qì* in the five *zàng* organs and below the heart as well as putrefaction in the mouth and bad breath; makes the teeth firm; brightens the eyes; and sharpens the ears. Consumed over a long time, it lightens the body and allows you to withstand aging. Grows in ponds and marshes in the far south.

續斷

一名龍豆，一名屬折
味苦，微溫，無毒

治傷寒，補不足，金瘡，癰傷，折跌，續筋骨，婦人乳難、崩中、漏血。久服益氣力。生山谷。

---

xùduàn

"reconnect what has been severed"
root of *Dipsacus asper* (teasel)
ALTERNATE NAMES: *lóngdòu* "dragon bean,"
shǔzhé "connecting breaks"
bitter flavor, slightly warm, non-toxic

Treats cold damage; supplements insufficiencies; [treats] incised wounds, damage from welling-abscesses, and fractures and falls; reconnects sinews and bones; and [treats] women's problems with breastfeeding and Center Flooding and spotting of blood. Consumed over a long time, it boosts qì and strength. Grows in mountain valleys.

漏蘆

一名野蘭
味苦,寒,無毒

治皮膚熱、惡瘡、疽、痔、濕痹,下乳汁。久服輕身,益氣,耳目聰明,不老,延年。生山谷。

---

lòulú

root of *Rhaponticum uniflorum* (globe thistle)
ALTERNATE NAME: *yělán* "wild orchid"
bitter flavor, cold, non-toxic

Treats heat in the skin, malign sores, flat-abscesses, Hemorrhoids, and damp-related *Bì* Impediment; and moves breast milk down. Consumed over a long time, it lightens the body, boosts qì, makes the ears and eyes sharp and bright, staves off aging, and extends the years. Grows in mountain valleys.

天名精

一名麥句薑,一名蝦蟆藍,一名豕首
味甘,寒,無毒

治瘀血、血瘕欲死,下血,止血,利小便,除小蟲,去痹,除胸中結熱,止煩渴。久服輕身,耐老。生平原、川澤。

---

tiānmíngjīng

"heaven name essence"
whole plant of *Carpesium abrotanoides* (carpesium)
ALTERNATE NAMES: *màigōujiāng* "wheat hook ginger,"
hámálán "frog indigo," *shǐshǒu* "boar's head"
sweet flavor, cold, non-toxic

Treats static blood and blood conglomerations that are life-threatening, moves the blood down, stops bleeding, disinhibits urine, gets rid of small worms, gets rid of *Bì* Impediment and binding heat inside the chest, and stops vexation with thirst. Consumed over a long time, it lightens the body and allows you to withstand aging. Grows in plains and in rivers and marshes.

決明子

味鹹,平,無毒

治青盲,目淫膚,赤白膜,眼赤痛,淚出。久服益精光,輕身。生川澤。

---

juémíngzi

"break through brightness seed"
seed of *Senna obtusifolia* (sicklepod, fetid cassia)
salty flavor, balanced, non-toxic

Treats Clear-eye Blindness, abnormal growth of tissue in the eyes, reddish-white membranes, redness and pain in the eyes, and tearing. Consumed over a long time, it boosts the essence brightness and lightens the body. Grows in rivers and marshes.

飛廉

一名飛輕
味苦,平,無毒

治骨節熱,脛重酸疼。久服令人身輕。生川澤。

---

fēilián

"fly into corners"
whole plant or root of *Carduus crispus* (welted thistle)
ALTERNATE NAME: *fēiqīng* "flying levity"
bitter flavor, balanced, non-toxic

Treats heat in the bones and joints and heaviness and soreness in the lower legs. Consumed over a long time, it makes your body light. Grows in rivers and marshes.

旋花

一名筋根花，一名金沸
味甘，溫，無毒

主益氣，去面䵟黑，色媚好。其根，味辛，治腹中寒熱邪氣，利小便。久服不饑，輕身。生平澤。

---

xuánhuā

"twirling flower"
flowers of *Calystegia sepium* (larger bindweed)
ALTERNATE NAMES: *jīngēnhuā* "sinew root flower,"
jīnfèi "metal froth"
sweet flavor, warm, non-toxic

Indicated for boosting qì, getting rid of spots and blackness in the face, and making the complexion alluring and beautiful. The root is acrid in flavor and treats the evil qì of cold and heat inside the abdomen and disinhibits urine. Consumed over a long time, it staves off hunger and lightens the body. Grows in marshy flatlands.

蘭草

一名水香
味辛,平,無毒

主利水道,殺蠱毒,辟不祥。久服益氣,輕身,不老,通神明。生池澤。

---

láncǎo

whole plant of *Eupatorium fortunei* (fragrant thoroughwort)
ALTERNATE NAME: *shuǐxiāng* "water fragrance"
acrid flavor, balanced, non-toxic

Indicated for disinhibiting the waterways, killing Gǔ Toxin, and warding off bad luck. Consumed over a long time, it boosts qì, lightens the body, staves off aging, and facilitates the breakthrough of spirit illumination. Grows in ponds and marshes.

蛇床子

一名蛇粟，一名蛇米
味苦，平，無毒

治婦人陰中腫痛，男子陰痿，濕癢，除痹氣，利關節，癲癇，惡瘡。久服輕身。生川谷及田野。

---

shéchuángzǐ

"snake bed seed"
fruit of *Cnidium monnieri* (cnidium seed)
ALTERNATE NAMES: *shésù* "snake millet,"
shémǐ "snake rice"
bitter flavor, balanced, non-toxic

Treats women's swelling and pain in the genitals and men's Yīn Wilt (i.e., impotence) and damp itch; gets rid of *Bì* Impediment qì; disinhibits the joints; and [treats] Epilepsy and malign sores. Consumed over a long time, it lightens the body. Grows in river valleys and in open fields.

地膚子

一名地葵
味苦,寒,無毒

治膀胱熱,利小便,補中,益精氣。久服耳目聰明,輕身,耐老。生平澤及田野。

---

dìfūzǐ

fruit of *Kochia scoparia* (summer cypress fruit)
ALTERNATE NAME: *dìkuí* "local mallow"
bitter flavor, cold, non-toxic

Treats heat in the bladder, disinhibits urine, supplements the center, and boosts essence qì. Consumed over a long time, it makes the ears and eyes sharp and bright, lightens the body, and allows you to withstand aging. Grows in marshy flatlands and in open fields.

景天

一名戒火,一名水母花,一名慎火
味苦,平,無毒

治大熱,火瘡,身熱,煩,邪惡氣。花,主女人漏下赤白,輕身,明目。生川谷。

---

jǐngtiān

"making heaven luminescent"
whole plant of *Sedum erythrosticum*[7] (stonecrop)
ALTERNATE NAMES: *jièhuǒ* "prohibit fire,"
shuǐmǔhuā "water mother flower," *shènhuǒ* "beware of fire"
bitter flavor, balanced, non-toxic

Treats great heat, fire wounds, generalized heat and vexation, and evil and malign qì. The flowers are indicated for women's vaginal spotting of red or white discharge, lightening the body, and brightening the eyes. Grows in river valleys.

茵陳蒿

味苦,平,無毒

治風濕寒熱邪氣,熱結,黃疸。久服輕身,益氣,耐老。生丘陵、坡岸上。

---

yīnchénhāo

whole plant of *Artemisia capillaris* or *scoparia*
(redstem or capillary wormwood)
bitter flavor, balanced, non-toxic

Treats the evil qì of wind, dampness, cold, or heat; heat bind; and jaundice. Consumed over a long time, it lightens the body, boosts qì, and allows you to withstand aging. Grows on hills and slopes.

杜若

一名杜蘅
味辛,微溫,無毒

治胸脅下逆氣,溫中,風入腦戶,頭腫痛,多涕,淚出。久服益精,明目,輕身。生川澤。

---

dùruò

rhizome and root, or whole plant of *Pollia japonica*
ALTERNATE NAME: *dùhéng*[8]
acrid flavor, slightly warm, non-toxic

Treats counterflow qì below the chest and rib-sides, warms the center, and [treats] wind entering through Nǎohù ("brain gate, DU-17"), swelling and pain in the head, copious snivel, and tearing. Consumed over a long time, it boosts essence, brightens the eyes, and lightens the body. Grows in rivers and marshes.

徐長卿

一名鬼督郵
味辛,溫,無毒

治鬼物百精,蠱毒,疫疾,邪惡氣,溫瘧。久服強悍,輕身。生山谷。

---

xúchángqīng

"staid leader of the stewards"
root of *Cynanchum paniculatum* (paniculate cynanchum)
ALTERNATE NAME: *guǐdūyóu* "demon inspector"[9]
acrid flavor, warm, non-toxic

Treats demonic entities and the hundred sprites, Gǔ Toxin, epidemics, evil and malign qì, and warm malaria. Consumed over a long time, it gives strength and valiance and lightens the body. Grows in mountain valleys.

石龍芻

一名龍鬚，一名草續斷，一名龍珠
味苦，微寒，無毒

治心腹邪氣，小便不利，淋閉，風濕，鬼疰，惡毒。久服補虛羸，輕身，耳目聰明，延年。生山谷濕地。

---

shílóngchú

"rock dragon hay"
whole herb of *Juncus effusus* (common rush)
ALTERNATE NAMES: *lóngxū* "dragon whiskers,"
cǎoxùduàn "field *xùduàn*," *lóngzhū* "dragon pearl"
bitter flavor, slightly cold, non-toxic

Treats evil qì in the heart and abdomen, inhibited urination, strangury and urinary block, wind and dampness, ghost infixation, and malign toxins. Consumed over a long time, it supplements emptiness and gauntness, lightens the body, makes the ears and eyes sharp and bright, and extends the years. Grows in mountain valleys in damp soil.

王不留行

味苦,平,無毒

治金瘡,止血,逐痛,出刺,除風痹、內寒。久服輕身,耐老,增壽。生山谷。

---

wángbùliúxíng

"the king does not detain advancement"
fruit of *Vaccaria hispanica/segetalis* (vaccaria)
bitter flavor, balanced, non-toxic

Treats incised wounds, stops bleeding, drives out pain, extrudes thorns, and gets rid of wind-related *Bì* Impediment and internal cold. Consumed over a long time, it lightens the body, allows you to withstand aging, and increases longevity. Grows in mountain valleys.

升麻

一名周麻
味甘、苦，平，無毒

主解百毒，殺百精、老物、殃鬼，辟溫疫、瘴氣、邪氣、蠱毒。久服不夭。生山谷。

---

shēngmá

rhizome of *Cimifuga foetida*, *dahurica*, or *heracleifolia*
(bugbane)
ALTERNATE NAME: *zhōumá* "Zhōu hemp"
sweet and bitter flavor, balanced, non-toxic

Indicated for resolving the hundred toxins; killing the hundred sprites, old entities, and calamitous ghosts; and warding off warm epidemics, miasmic qì, evil qì, and *Gǔ* Toxin. Consumed over a long time, it prevents premature death. Grows in mountain valleys.

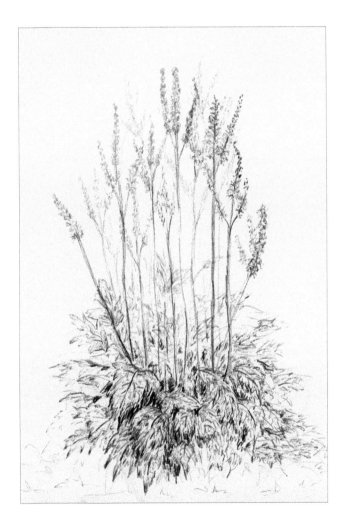

Sketch 9 - *shēngmá*

上藥

Upper Medicinals

木部

Trees

牡桂

味辛,溫,無毒

治上氣欬逆、結氣、喉痺、吐嘔,利關節,補中益氣。久服通神,輕身,不老。生南海山谷。

---

mǔguì

bark of *Cinnamomum cassia* (cinnamon)[10]
acrid flavor, warm, non-toxic

Treats counterflow cough with ascent of qì, bound qì, *Bì* Impediment in the throat, and vomiting and retching; disinhibits the joints; and supplements the center and boosts qì. Consumed over a long time, it facilitates the breakthrough of spirit [illumination], lightens the body, and staves off aging. Grows in mountain valleys in the far south.

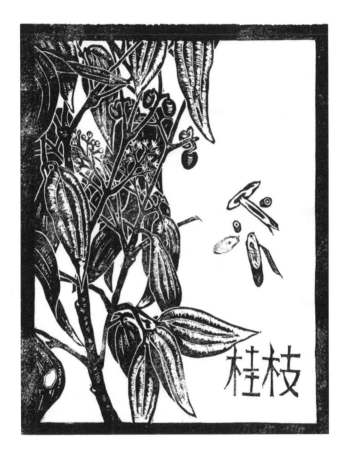

BLOCK PRINT 2 - *guìzhī*

菌桂

味辛,溫,無毒

治百病,養精神,和顏色,為諸藥先聘通使。久服輕身,不老,面生光華,媚好如童子。生山谷巖崖間。

---

jūnguì

bark of high-quality *Cinnamomum cassia*
(high-grade cinnamon)[11]
acrid flavor, warm, non-toxic

Treats the hundred diseases, nurtures the essence spirit(s), harmonizes the complexion, and serves as advance emissary for all sorts of medicinals. Consumed over a long time, it lightens the body, staves off aging, creates a brilliant glow on the face, and makes one beautiful and attractive like an adolescent. Grows in mountain valleys on rugged cliffs.

松脂

一名松膏,一名松肪
味苦,溫,無毒

治癰、疽、惡瘡、頭瘍、白禿、疥瘙、風氣,安五臟,除熱。久服輕身,不老,延年。生山谷。

sōngzhī

rosin of *Pinus massoniana* (pine rosin)
ALTERNATE NAMES: *sōnggāo* "pine salve,"
sōngfáng "pine lard"
bitter flavor, warm, non-toxic

Treats welling-abscesses, flat-abscesses, malign sores, open sores on the head, White Balding, itchy scabies with wind qì; calms the five *zàng* organs; and gets rid of heat. Consumed over a long time, it lightens the body, staves off aging, and extends the years. Grows in mountain valleys.

槐實

味苦,寒,無毒

治五內邪氣熱,止涎唾,補絕傷,五痔,火瘡,婦人乳瘕,子臟急痛。生平澤。

---

huáishí

fruit of *Sophora japonica* (pagoda tree fruit)
bitter flavor, cold, non-toxic

Treats evil qì and heat in the five internal [zàng organs]; stops drool and spittle; mends damage from severance; [treats] the five types of Hemorrhoids and fire wounds; and [treats] women's breast conglomerations, and tension and pain in the uterus. Grows in marshy flatlands.

枸杞

一名杞根,一名地骨,一名枸忌,一名地輔
味苦,寒,無毒

治五內邪氣,熱中,消渴,周痹。久服堅筋骨,輕身,不老。生平澤及諸丘陵阪岸。

---

gǒuqǐ

bark of the root[12] of *Lycium chinensis* (wolfsberry / goji)
ALTERNATE NAMES: *qǐgēn* "wolfberry root,"
dìgǔ "earth bone," *gōujì* "crooked dread,"
dìfǔ "earth buttress"
bitter flavor, cold, non-toxic

Treats evil qì in the five internal [*zàng* organs], "heat center/strike" [disease],[13] dispersion thirst, and pervasive *Bì* Impediment. Consumed over a long time, it makes the sinews and bones firm, lightens the body, and staves off aging. Grows in marshy flatlands, as well as, on all sorts of hills and slopes.

柏實

味甘,平,無毒

治驚悸,安五臟,益氣,除風濕痹。久服令人潤澤,美色,耳目聰明,不饑,不老,輕身,延年。生山谷。

---

bǎishí[14]

seed of *Platycladus orientalis* (arborvitae seed)
sweet flavor, balanced, non-toxic

Treats fright palpitations, calms the five *zàng* organs, boosts qì, and gets rid of wind- and damp-related *Bì* Impediment. Consumed over a long time, it allows you to become moist and lustrous, gives a lovely complexion, makes the ears and eyes sharp and bright, staves off hunger and aging, lightens the body, and extends the years. Grows in mountain valleys.

茯苓

一名茯菟
味甘，平，無毒

治胸脅逆氣、憂恚、驚邪、恐悸、心下結痛、寒熱、煩滿、欬逆，止口焦、舌乾，利小便。久服安魂魄，養神，不饑，延年。生山谷大松下。

---

fúlíng

"*fú* truffle"

dried fungus of *Wolfiporia extensa* or *Poria cocos* (China root)

ALTERNATE NAME: *fútù*

sweet flavor, balanced, non-toxic

Treats counterflow qì in the chest and rib-sides, worry and rage, fright evil, fear palpitations, binding and pain below the heart, cold and heat, vexation and fullness, cough with counterflow; stops parched mouth and dry tongue; and disinhibits urine. Consumed over a long time, it calms the *hún* and *pò* souls, nurtures the spirit(s), staves off hunger, and extends the years. Grows in mountain valleys below large pine trees.

榆皮

一名零榆
味甘,平,無毒

治大小便不通,利水道,除邪氣。久服輕身,不饑。其實尤良。生山谷。

---

yúpí

bark of *Ulmus pumila* (elm bark)
ALTERNATE NAME: *língyú* "drizzle elm"
sweet flavor, balanced, non-toxic

Treats clogged defecation and urination, disinhibits the waterways, and gets rid of evil qì. Consumed over a long time, it lightens the body and staves off hunger. The fruit is particularly good. Grows in mountain valleys.

酸棗

味酸,平,無毒

治心腹寒熱,邪結氣聚,四肢酸疼,濕痹。久服安五臟,輕身,延年。生川澤。

---

suānzǎo

fruit of *Ziziphus spinosa* (jujube)
sour flavor, balanced, non-toxic

Treats cold and heat in the heart and abdomen, evil binding and qì gathering, soreness in the four limbs, and damp-related *Bì* Impediment. Consumed over a long time, it calms the five *zàng* organs, lightens the body, and extends the years. Grows in rivers and marshes.

蔓荊實

味苦，微寒，無毒

治筋骨間寒熱、濕痹、拘攣，明目，堅齒，利九竅，去白蟲、長蟲。久服輕身，耐老。小荊實亦等。

---

mànjīngshí

fruit of *Vitex rotundifolia* (Vitex fruit)
bitter flavor, slightly cold, non-toxic

Treats cold and heat in the area of the sinews and bones, damp-related *Bì* Impediment, and hypertonicity; brightens the eyes; makes the teeth firm; disinhibits the Nine Orifices; and gets rid of white worms and long worms. Consumed over a long time, it lightens the body and allows you to withstand aging. *Xiǎojīngshí* is its equal.[15]

辛夷

一名辛矧,一名侯桃,一名房木
味辛,溫,無毒

治五臟身體寒熱,風頭,腦痛,面䵟。久服下氣,輕身,明目,增年,耐老。生川谷。

---

xīnyí

flower of *Magnolia liliflora/biondii/denudata* (magnolia)
ALTERNATE NAMES: *xīnshěn*, *hóutáo* "noble's peach,"
fángmù "building wood"
acrid flavor, warm, non-toxic

Treats cold and heat in the five *zàng* organs and in the torso and limbs, wind head, pain in the brain, and black spots in the face. Consumed over a long time, it brings down qì, lightens the body, brightens the eyes, increases the years, and allows you to withstand aging. Grows in river valleys.

五加皮

一名豺漆
味辛,溫,無毒

治心腹疝氣、腹痛,益氣,治躄、小兒不能行、疽瘡、陰蝕。

---

wǔjiāpí

"five additions bark"
root bark of *Eleutherococcus gracilistylus, sessiliflorus, senticosus, heryi,* or *verticillatus* [16] (acanthopanax bark)
ALTERNATE NAME: *cháiqī* "jackal lacquer"
acrid flavor, warm, non-toxic

Treats *shàn*-type ("mounding") qì in the heart and abdomen and abdominal pain; boosts qì; and treats lameness, small children's inability to walk, flat-abscesses, and genital erosion.

杜仲

一名思仙
味辛,平,無毒

治腰脊痛,補中,益精氣,堅筋骨,強志,除陰下癢濕、小便餘瀝。久服輕身,耐老。生山谷。

---

dùzhòng

bark of *Eucommia ulmoidis* (eucommia)
ALTERNATE NAME: *sīxiān* "thinking of transcendents"
acrid flavor, balanced, non-toxic

Treats lumbar and spinal pain, supplements the center, boosts essence qì, makes the sinews and bones firm, strengthens the will, and gets rid of damp itch below the genitals and lingering trickling of urine. Consumed over a long time, it lightens the body and allows you to withstand aging. Grows in mountain valleys.

女貞實

味苦,平,無毒

主補中,安五臟,養精神,除百病。久服肥健,輕身,不老。生川谷。

---

nǔzhēnshí

"female chastity seed"
fruit of *Ligustrum lucidum* (privet seed)
bitter flavor, balanced, non-toxic

Indicated for supplementing the center, calming the five *zàng* organs, nurturing the essence spirit(s), and getting rid of the hundred diseases. Consumed over a long time, it makes you plump and healthy, lightens the body, and staves off aging. Grows in river valleys.

蕤核

味甘,溫,無毒

治心腹邪結氣,明目,目赤痛傷,淚出。久服輕身,益氣,不饑,齆鼻。生川谷。

---

ruíhé[17]

seed of *Prinsepia uniflora*, (prinsepia seed)
sweet flavor, warm, non-toxic

Treats evil binding qì in the heart and abdomen, brightens the eyes, and [treats] redness, pain, and injury in the eyes, and tearing. Consumed over a long time, it lightens the body, boosts qì, staves off hunger, and [treats] nasal congestion. Grows in river valleys.

上藥

UPPER MEDICINALS

穀部

FOOD CROPS

橘柚

一名橘皮
味辛,溫,無毒

治胸中瘕熱、逆氣,利水穀。久服去口臭,下氣,通神明。生川谷。

---

júyòu

peel of *Citrus reticulata* (sour tangerine)
ALTERNATE NAME: *júpí* "tangerine peel"
acrid flavor, warm, non-toxic

Treats conglomerations, heat, and counterflow qì in the chest; and disinhibits solid and liquid food. Consumed over a long time, it gets rid of foul-smelling breath, brings down qì, and facilitates the breakthrough of spirit illumination. Grows in river valleys.

大棗

味甘,平,無毒

治心腹邪氣,安中養脾,助十二經,平胃氣,通九竅,補少氣、少津液、身中不足,大驚,四肢重,和百藥。久服輕身,長年。葉,覆麻黃能令出汗。生平澤。

---

dàzǎo

mature fruit of *Ziziphus jujuba* (jujube)
sweet flavor, balanced, non-toxic

Treats evil qì in the heart and abdomen; calms the center and nurtures the spleen; assists the twelve channels; levels stomach qì; unclogs the Nine Orifices; supplements shortage of qì and of fluids and insufficiency in the center of the body; [treats] great fright and heaviness of the four limbs; and harmonizes the hundred medicinals. Consumed over a long time, it lightens the body and lengthens the years. The leaves reinforce the ability of *máhuáng* to make the sweat come out. Grows in marshy flatlands.

葡萄

味甘,平,無毒

治筋骨濕痹,益氣,倍力,強志,令人肥健、耐饑、忍風寒。久食輕身,不老,延年。可作酒。生山谷。

---

pútáo

fruit of *Vitis vinifera* (grape)
sweet flavor, balanced, non-toxic

Treats damp-related *Bì* Impediment in the sinews and bones, boosts qì, multiplies strength, strengthens the will, makes you plump and healthy, and makes you withstand hunger and endure wind and cold. Eaten over a long time, it lightens the body, staves off aging, and extends the years. Can be turned into an alcoholic beverage. Grows in mountain valleys.

蓬蘽

一名覆盆
味酸，平，無毒

主安五臟，益精气，長陰令堅，强志，倍力，有子。久服輕身，不老。生平澤。

---

pénglěi

fruit of *Rubus tephrodes* (rubus)
ALTERNATE NAME: *fùpén* "overturned bowl"[18]
sour flavor, balanced, non-toxic

Indicated for calming the five *zàng* organs, boosting essence qì, lengthening the genitals and making them firm, strengthening the will, multiplying strength, and for fertility. Consumed over a long time, it lightens the body and staves off aging. Grows in marshy flatlands.

藕實莖

一名水芝
味甘,平,無毒

主補中,養神,益氣力,除百疾。久服輕身,耐老,不饑,延年。生池澤。

ǒushíjīng

seed and stalk of *Nelumbo nucifera* (lotus seed and stalk)
ALTERNATE NAME: *shuǐzhī* "water mushroom"
sweet flavor, balanced, non-toxic

Indicated for supplementing the center, nurturing the spirit(s), boosting qì and strength, and getting rid of the hundred acute diseases. Consumed over a long time, it lightens the body, allows you to withstand aging, staves off hunger, and extends the years. Grows in ponds and marshes.

雞頭實

一名雁喙實
味甘,平,無毒

治濕痹,腰脊膝痛,補中,除暴疾,益精氣,強志,令人耳目聰明。久服輕身,不饑,耐老,神仙。生池澤。

---

jītóushí

"chicken head seed"
seed of *Euryale ferox* (foxnut)
ALTERNATE NAME: *yànhuìshí* "goose-beak fruit"
sweet flavor, balanced, non-toxic

Treats damp-related *Bì* Impediment and pain in the lumbus, spine, and knees; supplements the center; gets rid of fulminant acute illnesses; boosts essence qì; strengthens the will; and allows your ears and eyes to be sharp and bright. Consumed over a long time, it lightens the body, staves off hunger, allows you to withstand aging, and [turns you into] a spirit immortal. Grows in ponds and marshes.

冬葵子

味甘,寒,無毒

治五臟六腑寒熱、羸瘦、五癃,利小便。久服堅骨,長肌肉,輕身,延年。

---

dōngkuízǐ

seed of *Malva verticillata* (mallow seed)
sweet flavor, cold, non-toxic

Treats cold and heat in the five *zàng* and six *fǔ* organs, gauntness, and the five types of dribbling urinary block; and disinhibits urine. Consumed over a long time, it makes the bones firm, grows the flesh, lightens the body, and extends the years.

莧實

一名馬莧
味甘,寒,無毒

治青盲,明目,除邪,利大小便,去寒熱。久服益氣力,不饑,輕身。生川澤及田中。

xiànshí

seed of *Amaranthus mangostanus* (amaranth seed)
ALTERNATE NAME: *mǎxiàn* "horse amaranth"
sweet flavor, cold, non-toxic

Treats Clear-eye Blindness, brightens the eyes, gets rid of evil, disinhibits urination and defecation, and gets rid of cold and heat. Consumed over a long time, it boosts qì and strength, staves off hunger, and lightens the body. Grows in rivers and marshes, as well as in the middle of fields.

白瓜子

一名水芝
味甘，平，無毒

主令人悦澤，好顏色，益氣，不饑。久服輕身，耐老。生平澤。

---

báiguāzǐ

"white gourd seed"
seed of *Benincasa hispida* (wax gourd seed)
ALTERNATE NAME: *shǔizhī* "water mushroom"
sweet flavor, balanced, non-toxic

Indicated for making you [appear] pleasing and lustrous, beautifying the complexion, boosting qì, and staving off hunger. Consumed over a long time, it lightens the body and allows you to withstand aging. Grows in marshy flatlands.

苦菜

一名荼草,一名選
味苦,寒,無毒

治五臟邪氣,厭穀,胃痹。久服安心,益氣,聰察,少臥,輕身,耐老。生川谷、山陵、道傍。

---

kǔcài

whole plant of *Sonchus oleraceus*
(sowthistle and similar bitter greens)[19]
ALTERNATE NAMES: *túcǎo* "sowthistle herb," *xuǎn* "to select"
bitter flavor, cold, non-toxic

Treats evil qì in the five *zàng* organs, loathing of solid foods, and *Bì* Impediment in the stomach. Consumed over a long time, it calms the heart, boosts qì, sharpens perspicacity, reduces [the need for] sleep, lightens the body, and allows you to withstand aging. Grows in river valleys, on hills, and alongside roads.

胡麻

一名巨勝，一名鴻藏
味甘，平，無毒

治傷中虛羸，補五內，益氣力，長肌肉，填髓腦。久服輕身，不老。生川澤。葉，名青蘘。味甘，寒，無毒。主五臟邪氣、風寒濕痹，益氣，補腦髓，堅筋骨。久服耳目聰明，不饑，不老，增壽。生川谷。

---

húmá

"barbarian hemp"
black seed of *Sesamum indicum* (black sesame)
ALTERNATE NAMES: *jùshèng* "immense victory,"
hóngzàng "swan treasury"
sweet flavor, balanced, non-toxic

Treats damage to the center with emptiness and gauntness, supplements the five internal [*zàng* organs], boosts qì and strength, grows flesh, and replenishes the marrow and brain. Consumed over a long time, it lightens the body and staves off aging. Grows in rivers and marshes. Leaves are called *qīngráng* ("blue-green wild ginger"). Sweet flavor, cold, non-toxic. Indicated for the evil qì of the five *zàng* organs; wind-, cold-, and damp-related *Bì* Impediment; boosting qì; supplementing the brain and marrow; and making the sinews and bones firm. Consumed over a long time, it makes the ears and eyes sharp and bright, staves off hunger and aging, and increases longevity. Grows in river valleys.

上藥

UPPER MEDICINALS

石部

ROCKS

丹砂

味甘,微寒,無毒。

治身體五臟百病,養精神,安魂魄,益氣,明目,殺精魅、邪惡鬼。久服通神明,不老。能化为汞。生山谷。

---

dānshā

cinnabar (mercuric sulfide)
sweet flavor, slightly cold, non-toxic

Treats the hundred diseases in the five *zàng* organs of the torso and extremities, nurtures the essence spirit(s), calms the *hún* and *pò* souls, boosts qì, brightens the eyes, and kills monsters, goblins, evil spirits, and malign ghosts. Consumed over a long time, it facilitates the breakthrough of spirit illumination and staves off aging. Can transform into mercury. Grows in mountain valleys.

雲母

一名雲珠，一名雲華，一名雲英，
一名雲液，一名雲砂，一名磷石
味甘，平，無毒

治身皮死肌、中風、寒熱、如在車船上，除邪氣，安五臟，益子精，明目。久服輕身，延年。生山谷山石間。

---

yúnmǔ

"cloud mother"

mica

ALTERNATE NAMES: *yúnzhū* "cloud pearl," *yúnhuá* "cloud flower," *yúnyīng* "cloud bloom," *yúnyè* "cloud secretion," *yúnshā* "cloud sand," *línshí* "phosphate rock"

sweet flavor, balanced, non-toxic

Treats dead flesh in the skin of the torso, being struck by wind, cold and heat, and [queasiness] as if [traveling] on a cart or boat; expels evil qì, calms the five *zàng* organs, boosts child essence, and brightens the eyes. Consumed over a long time, it lightens the body and extends the years. Grows in mountain valleys between mountain rocks.

玉泉

一名玉札
味甘，平，無毒

治五臟百病，柔筋，強骨，安魂魄，長肌肉，益氣。久服耐寒暑，不饑渴，不老，神仙。人臨死服五斤，死三年色不變。生山谷。

---

yùquán

"jade spring"
nephrite jade
ALTERNATE NAME: *yùzhá* "jade strip"
sweet flavor, balanced, non-toxic

Treats the hundred diseases of the five *zàng* organs, makes the sinews pliable, strengthens the bones, calms the *hún* and *pò* souls, lengthens the flesh, and boosts qì. Consumed over a long time, it allows you to withstand cold and summer-heat, staves off hunger and thirst, staves off aging, and [makes you] a spirit-immortal. If a person ingests five *jīn* ("catties") when they are just about to die, three years after death the complexion will remain unchanged. Grows in mountain valleys.

石鐘乳

一名留公乳
味甘,溫,無毒

治欬逆上氣,明目,益精,安五臟,通百節,利九竅,下乳汁。生山谷。

---

shízhōngrǔ

"rock bell breast"
stalactite
ALTERNATE NAME: *liúgōngrǔ* "lingering old man breast"
sweet flavor, warm, non-toxic

Treats counterflow cough with ascent of qì, brightens the eyes, boosts essence, calms the five *zàng* organs, unclogs the hundred joints, disinhibits the Nine Orifices, and brings down the breast milk. Grows in mountain valleys.

礬石

一名羽涅
味酸,寒,無毒

治寒熱、泄利、白沃、陰蝕、惡瘡、目痛,堅骨齒。煉餌服之,輕身,不老,增年。生山谷。

---

fánshí

alum

ALTERNATE NAME: *yǔniè* "plumed sludge"
sour flavor, cold, non-toxic

Treats cold and heat, diarrhea, white soaking [i.e., white vaginal discharge], genital erosion, malign sores, and eye pain; and makes the bones and teeth firm. Consumed as an alchemically refined substance, it lightens the body, staves off aging, and increases the years. Grows in mountain valleys.

消石

一名芒消
味苦,寒,無毒

治五臟積熱、胃脹閉,滌去蓄結飲食,推陳致新,除邪氣。煉之如膏,久服輕身。生山谷。

---

xiāoshí

"dissolving rock"
niter/saltpeter
ALTERNATE NAME: *mángxiāo* [20] (refined mirabilite)
bitter flavor, cold, non-toxic

Treats accumulated heat in the five *zàng* organs, and distention and blockage in the stomach; flushes out amassed and bound food and drink; pushes out the old and institutes the new; and expels evil qì. Refined into a paste-like substance and consumed over a long time, it lightens the body. Grows in mountain valleys.

朴消

味苦，寒，無毒

治百病，除寒熱邪氣，逐六腑積聚、結固、留癖，能化七十二種石。煉餌服之，輕身，神仙。生山谷，有鹹水之陽。

---

pòxiāo

unrefined mirabilite
bitter flavor, cold, non-toxic

Treats the hundred diseases; expels the evil qì of cold and heat; drives out accumulations and gatherings in the six *fǔ* organs, bound and fixed [masses], and lingering *Pǐ* Aggregations; and is able to transform the seventy-two types of rocks. Consumed as an alchemically refined substance, it lightens the body and [makes you] a spirit immortal. Grows in mountain valleys and possesses the yáng of salt water.

滑石

味甘，寒，無毒

治身熱、泄辟、女子乳難、癃閉，利小便，蕩胃中積聚、寒熱，益精氣。久服輕身，耐饑，長年。生山谷。

---

huáshí

"slippery rock"
talcum/soapstone
sweet flavor, cold, non-toxic

Treats generalized fever, diarrhea and [intestinal] afflux, women's problems with breastfeeding, and dribbling urinary block; disinhibits urine; flushes out accumulations and gatherings and heat and cold from inside the stomach; and boosts essence qì. Consumed over a long time, it lightens the body, allows you to withstand hunger, and lengthens the years. Grows in mountain valleys.

空青

味甘，寒，無毒

治青盲、耳聾，明目，利九竅，通血脉，養精神。久服輕身，延年，不老。能化銅、鐵、鉛、錫作金。生山谷有銅處。

---

kōngqīng

hollow azure
hollow azurite
sweet flavor, cold, non-toxic

Treats Clear-eye Blindness and deafness, brightens the eyes, disinhibits the Nine Orifices, unclogs the blood vessels, and nurtures the essence spirit(s). Consumed over a long time, it lightens the body, extends the years, and staves off aging. Able to transform copper, iron, lead, and tin into gold. Grows in mountain valleys in locations where there is copper.

曾青

味酸,小寒,無毒

治目痛,止淚出、風痹,利關節,通九竅,破癥堅積聚。久服輕身,不老,能化金、銅。生山谷。

---

céngqīng

layered azure
layered azurite
sour flavor, mildly cold, non-toxic

Treats eye pain; stops tears from emerging and wind *Bì* Impediment; disinhibits the joints; unclogs the Nine Orifices; and breaks up concretions, hardenings, accumulations, and gatherings. Consumed over a long time, it lightens the body, staves off aging, and is able to transform gold and copper. Grows in mountain valleys.

禹餘糧

一名白餘糧
味甘,寒,無毒

治欬逆,寒熱,煩滿,下利赤白,血閉,癥瘕,大熱。煉餌服之,不饑,輕身,延年。生東海、池澤及山島中。

---

yǔyúliáng

sea limonite
ALTERNATE NAME: *báiyúliáng* "white *yúliáng*"
sweet flavor, cold, non-toxic

Treats counterflow cough, cold and heat, vexation and fullness, red and white diarrhea, blood block, concretions and conglomerations, and severe heat. Consumed as an alchemically refined substance, it staves off hunger, lightens the body, and extends the years. Grows in the East China Sea,[21] in ponds and marshes, and on mountainous islands.

太一餘糧

一名石腦
味甘,平,無毒

治欬逆上氣、癥瘕、血閉、漏下,除邪氣。久服耐寒暑,不饑,輕身,飛行千里,神仙。生山谷。

---

tàiyīyúliáng

mountain limonite[22]
ALTERNATE NAME: *shínǎo* "rock brain"
sweet flavor, balanced, non-toxic

Treats counterflow cough with ascent of qì, concretions and conglomerations, blood block, and vaginal spotting; and expels evil qì. Consumed over a long time, it allows you to withstand cold and summer-heat, staves off hunger, lightens the body, allows you to fly a thousand miles, and turns you into a spirit immortal. Grows in mountain valleys.

白石英

味甘,微溫,無毒

治消渴、陰痿不足、欬逆、胸膈間久寒,益氣,除風濕痹。久服輕身,長年。生山谷。

---

báishíyīng

"white rock bloom"
white quartz
sweet flavor, slightly warm, non-toxic

Treats dispersion thirst, Yīn Wilt (i.e. impotence) and [sexual] insufficiency, counterflow cough, and chronic cold in the area of the chest and diaphragm; boosts qì; and gets rid of wind- and damp-related *Bì* Impediment. Consumed over a long time, it lightens the body and lengthens the years. Grows in mountain valleys.

紫石英

味甘,溫,無毒

治心腹欬逆、邪氣,補不足,女子風寒在子宮,絕孕,十年無子。久服溫中,輕身,延年。生山谷。

---

zǐshíyīng[23]

"purple rock bloom"
fluorite
sweet flavor, warm, non-toxic

Treats counterflow cough and evil qì in the heart and abdomen; supplements insufficiencies; and [treats] the presence of women's wind and cold in the uterus, interrupted pregnancies, and infertility for ten years. Consumed over a long time, it warms the center, lightens the body, and extends the years. Grows in mountain valleys.

青石脂

味甘,平,無毒

主養肝膽氣,治黃疸、瀉利、腸澼及疽、痔、惡瘡。久服補髓,益氣,不饑,延年。生山谷中。

---

qīngshízhī

"azure rock grease"
green-blue clay
sweet flavor, balanced, non-toxic

Indicated for nurturing the qì of the liver and gallbladder and treating jaundice, diarrhea, intestinal afflux and flat-abscesses, Hemorrhoids, and malign sores. Consumed over a long time, it supplements the marrow, boosts qì, staves off hunger, and extends the years. Grows in the center of mountain valleys.

赤石脂

味甘,平,無毒

主養心氣,下利赤白,小便利及癰、疽、瘍、痔。久服補髓,益智,輕身,延年。生山谷中。

---

chìshízhī[24]

"red rock grease"
red clay
sweet flavor, balanced, non-toxic

Indicated for nurturing the qì of the heart, for red and white diarrhea, and for disinhibited urination and welling- and flat-abscesses, sores, and hemorrhoids. Consumed over a long time, it supplements the marrow, boosts wisdom, lightens the body, and extends the years. Grows in the center of mountain valleys.

黃石脂

味甘,平,無毒

主養脾氣,大人、小兒泄利,腸澼,下膿血,除黃疸。久服輕身,延年。生山谷中。

---

huángshízhī

"yellow rock grease"
yellow clay
sweet flavor, balanced, non-toxic

Indicated for nurturing the qì of the spleen, for diarrhea in both adults and young children, for intestinal afflux, and for moving pus and blood down [and out of the body] and getting rid of jaundice. Consumed over a long time, it lightens the body and extends the years. Grows in the center of mountain valleys.

白石脂

味甘,平,無毒

主養肺氣,補骨髓,排癰、疽、瘡、痔。久服不饑,輕身,長年。生山谷中。

---

báishízhī

"white rock grease"
white clay
sweet flavor, balanced, non-toxic

Indicated for nurturing the qì of the lung, supplementing the bone and marrow, and pushing out welling- and flat-abscesses, sores, and Hemorrhoids. Consumed over a long time, it staves off hunger, lightens the body, and lengthens the years. Grows in the center of mountain valleys.

黑石脂

一名石涅，一名石墨
味甘，平，無毒

主養腎氣，強陰，治陰蝕瘡，止腸澼、泄利。久服益氣，不饑，延年。生山谷中。

---

hēishízhī

"black rock grease"
black clay
ALTERNATE NAMES: *shínìe* "rock sludge," *shímò* "rock ink"
sweet flavor, balanced, non-toxic

Indicated for nurturing the qì of the kidney, strengthening yīn, treating genital erosion sores, and stopping intestinal afflux and diarrhea. Consumed over a long time, it boosts qì, staves off hunger, and extends the years. Grows in the center of mountain valleys.

白青

味甘,平,無毒

主明目,利九竅,耳聾,心下邪氣,令人吐,殺諸毒、三蟲。久服通神明,輕身,延年,不老。生山谷。

---

báiqīng

"white azurite"[25]
sweet flavor, balanced, non-toxic

Indicated for brightening the eyes, disinhibiting the Nine Orifices, for deafness and evil qì below the heart, for inducing vomiting, and for killing all sorts of toxins and the Three Worms. Consumed over a long time, it facilitates the breakthrough of spirit illumination, lightens the body, extends the years, and staves off aging. Grows in mountain valleys.

扁青

味甘,平,無毒

治目痛、明目、折跌、癰腫、金瘡不瘳,破積聚,解毒氣,利精神。久服輕身,不老。生山谷。

---

biǎnqīng

"flat azurite"[26]
sweet flavor, balanced, non-toxic

Treats eye pain; brightens the eyes; [treats] breaks and falls, welling-abscesses with swelling, and incised wounds that fail to heal; breaks up accumulations and gatherings; resolves toxic qì; and disinhibits the essence spirit(s). Consumed over a long time, it lightens the body and staves off aging. Grows in mountain valleys.

上藥

Upper Medicinals

蟲部

Insects

龍骨

味甘,平,無毒

治心腹鬼疰,精物老魅,欬逆,泄利膿血,女子漏下,癥瘕堅結,小兒熱氣驚癇。龍齒,平。治小兒、大人驚癇,癲疾,狂走,心下結氣,不能喘息,諸痙,殺精物。久服輕身,通神明,延年。生川谷及巖水岸土穴中死龍處。

lónggǔ

"dragon bones"
fossil bones
sweet flavor, balanced, non-toxic

Treats demonic infixation in the heart and abdomen, spectral entities and old evil sprites, counterflow cough, diarrhea with pus and blood, women's vaginal spotting, concretions and conglomerations, hardenings and binds, and heat qì and fright Seizures in small children. Dragon teeth: balanced. Indicated for fright

Seizures in small children and adults, withdrawal disease, manic running, bound qì below the heart, inability to pant and breathe, and all sorts of tetany, and for killing spectral entities. Consumed over a long time, it lightens the body, facilitates the breakthrough of spirit illumination, and extends the years. Grows in river valleys and in places where dragons have died inside earthen caves in cliffs and coastal and river embankments.

熊脂

一名熊白
味甘,微寒,無毒

治風痹不仁,筋急,五臟腹中積聚,寒熱,羸瘦,頭瘍,白禿,面䵟皰。久服強志,不饑,輕身。生山谷。

---

xióngzhī

bear fat

ALTERNATE NAME: *xióngbái* "bear's white"
sweet flavor, slightly cold, non-toxic

Treats wind-related *Bì* Impediment and numbness, hypertonicity in the sinews, accumulations and gatherings in the five *zàng* organs and inside the abdomen, cold and heat, gauntness, open sores on the head, White Balding, and black spots and blisters on the face. Consumed over a long time, it strengthens the will, staves off hunger, and lightens the body. Grows in mountain valleys.

白膠

一名鹿角膠
味甘，平，無毒

治傷中，勞絕，腰痛，羸瘦，補中益氣，婦人血閉，無子，止痛，安胎。久服輕身，延年。

---

báijiāo

"white glue"
deer antler glue
ALTERNATE NAME: *lùjiǎojiāo* "deer horn glue"
sweet flavor, balanced, non-toxic

Treats damage to the center, taxation-related expiry, lumbar pain, and gauntness; supplements the center and boosts qì; and [and is indicated for treating] women's blood block and infertility, stopping pain, and quieting the fetus. Consumed over a long time, it lightens the body and extends the years.

阿膠

一名傅致膠
味甘，平，無毒

治心腹內崩、勞極、灑灑如瘧狀、腰腹痛、四肢酸疼、女子下血，安胎。久服輕身、益氣。

ējiāo

donkey hide glue
ALTERNATE NAME: *fùzhìjiāo*
sweet flavor, balanced, non-toxic

Treats internal flooding in the heart or abdomen, culminating taxation, shivering like in malaria, lumbar and abdominal pain, soreness and pain in the four limbs, and women's vaginal bleeding; and quiets the fetus. Consumed over a long time, it lightens the body and boosts qì.

丹雄雞

一名載丹
味甘，微溫，無毒

治女人崩中、漏下、赤白沃，補虛，溫中，止血，通神，殺毒，辟不祥。頭，主殺鬼，東門上者尤良。肪，治耳聾。腸，治遺溺。肶胵裏黃皮，治泄利。屎白，治消渴，傷寒，寒熱。黑雌雞，治風寒濕痹、溫、五緩、六急，安胎。翮羽，主下血閉。雞子，主除熱、火瘡、癇、痓，可作琥珀神物。雞白蠹，能肥豬。生平泽。

---

dānxióngjī

"cinnabar-red rooster"
ALTERNATE NAME: *zàidān* "loaded with cinnabar"
sweet flavor, slightly warm, non-toxic

Treats women's Center Flooding, vaginal spotting, and red and white soaking; supplements emptiness; warms the center; stops bleeding; facilitates the breakthrough of spirit illumination; kills toxins; and wards off bad luck.[27] The head is indicated for killing ghosts, with one from above the eastern gate being particularly good. The fat treats deafness. The intestines treat enuresis. The yellow skin from inside the gizzard treats diarrhea. The white in the excrement treats dispersion thirst, cold damage, and cold and heat. Black hen treats wind-, cold-, and damp-related *Bì* Impediment, [pathogenic] warmth, the five types of hypotonicity and six types of hypertonicity; and quiets the fetus. The feathers are indicated for moving down blood block. The eggs are indicated for getting rid of heat, burns, Seizures, and tetany, and can produce the divine substance amber. The white open-ended sack of the chicken[28] is able to fatten pigs. Grows in marshy flatlands.

雁肪

一名鶩肪
味甘,平,無毒

治風攣拘急,偏枯,氣不通利。肉,味甘,平,無毒。久服長毛髮鬚眉,益氣,不饑,輕身,耐老。生池澤。

---

yànfáng

goose fat

ALTERNATE NAME: *wùfáng* "duck fat"
sweet flavor, balanced, non-toxic

Treats wind-related contractions and hypertonicity, hemilateral withering, and failure of the qì to move freely. The flesh is sweet in flavor, balanced, and non-toxic. Consumed over a long time, it makes the body hair, head hair, beard, and eyebrows grow; boosts qì; staves off hunger; lightens the body; and allows you to withstand aging. Grows in ponds and marshes.

石蜜

一名石飴
味甘,平,無毒

治心腹邪氣、諸驚癇痙,安五臟,諸不足,益氣補中,止痛,解毒,除眾病,和百藥。久服強志,輕身,不饑,不老。生山谷及諸山石中。

---

shímì

honey

ALTERNATE NAME: *shíyí* "rock candy"
sweet flavor, balanced, non-toxic

Treats evil qì in the heart and abdomen, all sorts of fright Seizures and tetany; calms the five *zàng* organs; [treats] all sorts of insufficiencies; boosts qì and supplements the center; stops pain; resolves toxins; gets rid of the multitudes of diseases; and harmonizes the hundred medicinals. Consumed over a long time, it strengthens the will, lightens the body, and staves off hunger and aging. Grows in mountain valleys and inside all sorts of mountain rocks.

蜂子

一名蜚零
味甘,平,無毒

治頭風,除蠱毒,補虛羸,傷中。久服令人光澤,好顏色,不老。大黃蜂子,主心腹脹滿痛,輕身,益氣。土蜂子,平,治癰腫。生山谷。

---

fēngzǐ

wasp

ALTERNATE NAME: *fěilíng*

sweet flavor, balanced, non-toxic

Treats head wind, expels *Gǔ* Toxins, supplements emptiness and gauntness, and [treats] damage to the center. Consumed over a long time, it makes you lustrous, beautifies the complexion, and staves off aging. The Large Yellow Wasp is indicated for distention, fullness, and pain in the heart and abdomen; lightening the body; and boosting qì. The Wild Wasp is balanced and treats welling-abscesses with swelling. Grows in mountain valleys.

蜜蠟

味甘,微溫,無毒

治下利膿血,補中,續絕傷,金瘡,益氣。不饑,耐老。生山谷蜜房、木石間。

---

mìlà

beeswax
sweet flavor, slightly warm, non-toxic

Treats diarrhea with pus and blood, supplements the center, reconnects damage from severance, [treats] incised wounds, and boosts qì. Staves off hunger and allows you to withstand aging. Grows in hives in mountain valleys and in trees and rocks.

牡蠣

一名蠣蛤
味鹹，平，無毒

治傷寒寒熱、溫虐灑灑、驚恚怒氣，除拘緩、鼠瘻、女子帶下赤白。久服強骨節，杀鬼，延年。生東海池澤。

---

mǔlì

oyster shell

ALTERNATE NAME: *lìgé*

salty flavor, balanced, non-toxic

Treats cold damage with cold and heat, warm malaria with shivering, and fright, rage, and angry qì; gets rid of [alternating] tensing and slackening; and [treats] Rat Fistulas and women's vaginal discharge in red or white. Consumed over a long time, it strengthens the bones and joints, kills ghosts, and extends the years. Grows in the East China Sea and in ponds and marshes.

中藥
MIDDLE MEDICINALS

草部
HERBS

乾薑

味辛,溫,無毒

治胸滿,欬逆上氣,溫中,止血,出汗,逐風,濕痹,腸澼下痢。生者尤良。味辛,微溫。久服去臭氣,通神明。生川谷。

---

gānjiāng

dried root of *Zingiber officinale* (dried ginger)
acrid flavor, warm, non-toxic

Treats fullness in the chest and counterflow cough with ascent of qì, warms the center, stops bleeding, promotes sweating, drives out wind, [and treats] damp-related *Bì* Impediment and intestinal afflux and diarrhea. The fresh [root] is particularly excellent. It is acrid in flavor and slightly warm. Consumed over a long time, it gets rid of foul smells and facilitates the breakthrough of spirit illumination. Grows in river valleys.

葈耳實

一名胡葈，一名地葵
味甘，溫，有小毒

治風頭寒痛，風濕周痹，四肢拘攣痛，惡肉死肌。久服益氣，耳目聰明，強志，輕身。生川谷及田野。

---

xǐěrshí

fruit of *Xanthium sibiricum* (cocklebur)[1]
ALTERNATE NAME: *húxǐ* "Western cocklebur,"
dìkuí "native mallow"
sweet flavor, warm, slightly toxic

Treats wind head with cold pain, pervasive wind- and damp-related *bì* impediment, hypertonicity of the four limbs, and malign and dead flesh. Consumed over a long time, it boosts qì, makes the ears and eyes sharp and bright, strengthens the will, and lightens the body. Grows in river valleys and open fields.

葛根

一名雞齊根
味甘,平,無毒

治消渴、身大熱、嘔吐、諸痺,起陰氣,解諸毒。葛穀,治下利十歲以上。生川谷。

---

gégēn

root of *Pueraria lobata*[2] (kudzu)
ALTERNATE NAME: *jīqígēn* "chicken Qí root"
sweet flavor, balanced, non-toxic

Treats dispersion thirst, great heat in the body, retching and vomiting, and all sorts of *Bì* Impediment; lifts up yīn qì; and resolves all sorts of toxins. The seed treats diarrhea in patients [that has persisted] for more than ten years. Grows in river valleys.

栝樓根

一名地樓
味苦,寒,無毒

治消渴、身熱、煩滿、大熱,補虛,安中,續絕傷。生川谷及山陰地。

---

guālóugēn

root of *Trichosanthes kirilowii* (wild snake gourd)
ALTERNATE NAME: *dìlóu* "native gourd"[3]
bitter flavor, cold, non-toxic

Treats dispersion thirst, generalized heat, vexation and fullness, and great heat; supplements emptiness; calms the center; and reconnects damage from severance. Grows in river valleys and in shady ground on mountains.

苦參

一名水槐,一名苦蘵
味苦,寒,無毒

治心腹結氣、癥瘕積聚、黃疸、溺有餘瀝,逐水,除癰腫,補中,明目,止淚。生山谷及田野。

kǔshēn

"bitter *shēn*"
root of *Sophora flavescens* (sophora)
ALTERNATE NAMES: *shuǐhuái* "water sophora," *kǔshí*
bitter flavor, cold, non-toxic

Treats bound qì in the heart and abdomen, concretions, conglomerations, accumulations, and gatherings, jaundice, and lingering dripping after urination; drives out water; gets rid of welling-abscesses with swelling; supplements the center; brightens the eyes; and stops tearing. Grows in mountain valleys and open fields.

芎藭

味辛,溫,無毒

治中風入腦,頭痛,寒痹,筋攣緩急,金瘡,婦人血閉,無子。生川谷。

---

xiōngqióng

rhizome of *Ligusticum wallichii* (*chuānxiōng* lovage)
acrid flavor, warm, non-toxic

Treats wind strike entering the brain, headache, cold-related *Bì* Impediment, contraction of the sinews and slackening and tensing, incised wounds, blood block in women, and infertility. Grows in river valleys.

當歸

一名乾歸
味甘,溫,無毒

治欬逆上氣,溫瘧,寒熱洗洗在皮膚中,婦人漏下、絕子,諸惡瘡瘍,金瘡。煮飲之。生川谷。

---

dāngguī

"should return home"
root of *Angelica sinensis* or *polymorpha*
(Chinese angelica)
ALTERNATE NAME: *gānguī* "dry return home"
sweet flavor, warm, non-toxic

Treats counterflow cough with ascent of qì, warm malaria, cold and heat with shivering inside the skin, vaginal leaking and interrupted childbearing in women, all sorts of malign sores and festering ulcers, and incised wounds. Decoct it and drink it. Grows in river valleys.

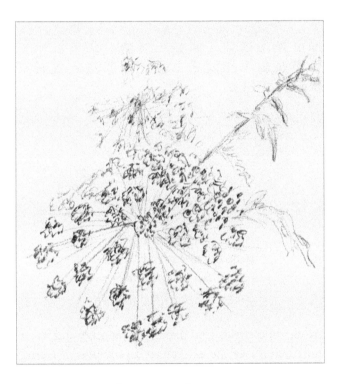

Sketch 10 - *dāngguī*

麻黃

一名龍沙
味甘，溫，無毒

治中風、傷寒、頭痛、溫瘧，發表出汗，去邪熱氣，止欬逆上氣，除寒熱，破癥堅積聚。生川谷。

---

máhuáng

"hemp yellow"
stalks of *Ephedra sinica* (ephedra)
ALTERNATE NAME: *lóngshā* "dragon sand"
sweet flavor, warm, non-toxic

Treats wind strike, cold damage, headache, and warm malaria; effuses the exterior and promotes sweating; gets rid of evil heat qì; stops counterflow cough with ascent of qì; expels cold and heat; and breaks up concretions, firmness, accumulations, and gatherings. Grows in river valleys.

通草

一名附支
味辛,平,無毒

主去惡蟲,除脾胃寒熱,通利九竅、血脈、關節,令人不忘。生山谷及山陽。

---

tōngcǎo

"unclogging herb"
pith in the stalk of *Tetrapanax papyrifera* (rice-paper plant)
ALTERNATE NAME: *fùzhī* "adjoining branch"
acrid flavor, balanced, non-toxic

Indicated for getting rid of malign worms and of cold and heat in the spleen and stomach, unclogging the Nine Orifices, blood vessels, and joints, and staving off forgetfulness. Grows in mountain valleys and on the south-facing side of mountains.

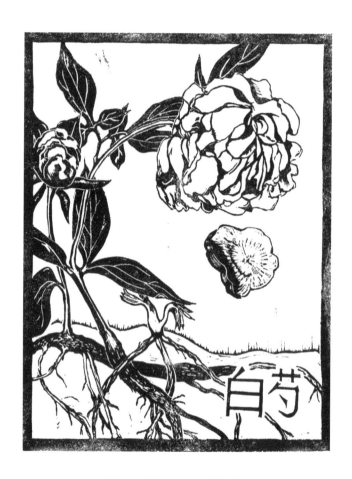

Block Print 3 - *sháoyào*

芍藥

一名白朮
味苦，平，有小毒

治邪氣腹痛，除血痹，破堅積，寒熱，疝瘕，止痛，利小便，益氣。生川谷及丘陵。

---

sháoyào

root of *Paeonia lactiflora* (peony)
ALTERNATE NAME: *báimù* "white wood"
bitter flavor, balanced, slightly toxic

Treats evil qì with abdominal pain, gets rid of blood *Bì* Impediment, breaks up firmness and accumulations, [treats] cold and heat and *shàn*-type ("mounding") conglomerations, stops pain, disinhibits urination, and boosts qì. Grows in river valleys and on hills.

蠡實

一名劇草，一名三堅，一名豕首
味甘，平，無毒

治皮膚寒熱、胃中熱氣、風寒濕痺，堅筋骨，令人嗜食。久服輕身。花、葉，去白蟲、喉痺。生川谷。

---

líshí[4]

seed of *Iris Pallasii* (North China iris)
ALTERNATE NAMES: *jùcǎo* "intense herb,"
sānjiān "triple firmness," *shǐshǒu* "pig's head"[5]
sweet flavor, balanced, non-toxic

Treats cold and heat in the skin, hot qì inside the stomach, and wind-, cold-, and damp-related *Bì* Impediment; makes the sinews and bones firm; and causes you to crave food. Consumed over a long time, it lightens the body. The flowers and leaves get rid of white worms and *Bì* Impediment in the throat. Grows in river valleys.

瞿麥

一名巨句麥
味苦，寒，無毒

治關格、諸癃結、小便不通，出刺，決癰腫，明目，去翳，破胎墮子，下閉血。生川谷。

qúmài

"panic wheat"

whole plant of *Dianthus superbus* or *chinensis* (dianthus)

ALTERNATE NAME: *jùjùmài* "huge phrase wheat"

bitter flavor, cold, non-toxic

Treats Barrier Repulsion, all forms of dribbling urinary stoppages (*lóng*) and binding, and clogged urination; makes thorns come out; bursts welling-abscesses with swelling; brightens the eyes; gets rid of eye screens; breaks up fetuses and causes them to drop;[6] and brings down blocked blood. Grows in river valleys.

玄參

一名重臺
味苦,微寒,無毒

治腹中寒熱積聚、女子產乳餘疾,補腎氣,令人目明。生川谷。

---

xuánshēn

"dark *shēn*"
root of Scrophularia ningpoensis (figwort)
ALTERNATE NAME: *chóngtái* "double-petaled flower"
bitter flavor, slightly cold, non-toxic

Treats cold and heat and accumulations and gatherings inside the abdomen, and women's residual diseases after childbearing and breastfeeding; supplements kidney qì; and makes a person's eyes bright. Grows in river valleys.

秦艽

一名秦瓜
味苦,平,無毒

治寒熱邪氣、寒濕風痹、肢節痛,下水,利小便。生川谷。

---

qínjiāo

root of *Gentiana macrophylla* (large-leaved gentian)
ALTERNATE NAME: *qínguā* "Qín melon"
bitter flavor, balanced, non-toxic

Treats evil qì of cold and heat, cold-, damp-, and wind-related *Bì* Impediment, and pain in the joints of the limbs; moves water down; and disinhibits urination. Grows in river alleys.

百合

味甘,平,無毒

治邪氣腹脹、心痛,利大小便,補中益氣。生山谷。

---

bǎihé

"hundred union"
bulb of *Lilium lancifolium*[7] (lily)
sweet flavor, balanced, non-toxic

Treats evil qì abdominal distention and heart pain, disinhibits defecation and urination, and supplements the center and boosts qì. Grows in mountain valleys.

知母

一名蚳母,一名連母,一名野蓼,
一名地參,一名水參,一名水浚,
一名貨母,一名蝭母
味苦,寒,無毒

治消渴、熱中,除邪氣、肢體浮腫,下水,補不足,益氣。生川谷

---

zhīmǔ

"mother of knowing"
rhizome of *Anemarrhena asphodeloides* (anemarrhena)
ALTERNATE NAMES: *chímǔ* "green-frog mother,"
liánmǔ "linking mother," *yěliáo* "wild wasteland,"
dìshēn "native shēn," *shuǐshēn* "water shēn,"
shuǐjùn "water dredging," *huòmǔ* "mother of wealth,"
tímǔ "cicada mother"
bitter flavor, cold, non-toxic

Treats dispersion thirst and heat in the center, expels evil qì and superficial swelling in the limbs and body, moves water down, supplements insufficiency, and boosts qì. Grows in river valleys.

貝母

一名空草
味辛,平,無毒

治傷寒煩熱,淋瀝邪氣,疝瘕,喉痹,乳難,金瘡,風痙。

---

bèimǔ

"mother of conch"
bulb of *Fritillaria cirrhosa* (fritillary)
ALTERNATE NAME: *kōngcǎo* "empty herb"
acrid flavor, balanced, non-toxic

Treats cold damage with heat vexation, the evil qì of strangury and dribbling, *shàn*-type ("mounding") conglomerations, *Bì* Impediment in the throat, lactation problems, incised wounds, and wind Seizures.

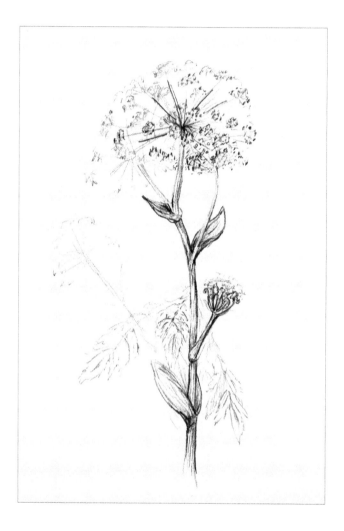

SKETCH 11 - *báizhǐ*

白芷

一名芳香
味辛,溫,無毒

治女人漏下赤白、血閉、陰腫,寒熱,風頭侵目淚出。長肌膚,潤澤,可作面脂。生川谷下澤。

---

báizhǐ

root of *Angelica dahurica* (Dahurian angelica)
ALTERNATE NAME: *fāngxiāng* "aromatic fragrance"
acrid flavor, warm, non-toxic

Treats women's vaginal spotting in red or white, blood block, and genital swelling; cold and heat; and wind in the head invading the eyes and causing tearing. Makes the skin and flesh grow, moistens and lubricates, and can be used as an ointment for the face. Grows in river valleys and low-lying marshes.

淫羊藿

一名剛前
味辛,寒,無毒

治陰痿、絕傷、莖中痛,利小便,益氣力,強志。生山谷。

---

yínyánghuò

"lascivious goat pulse"
whole plant of *Epimedium grandiflorum* (barrenwort)
ALTERNATE NAME: *gāngqián* "rigid anterior"
acrid flavor, cold, non-toxic

Treats Yīn Wilt, damage from severance, and pain inside the penis; disinhibits urination; boosts qì and strength, and strengthens the will. Grows in mountain valleys.

黃芩

一名腐腸
味苦，平，無毒

治諸熱、黃疸、腸澼、泄利，逐水，下血閉，惡瘡疽蝕，火瘍。生川谷。

---

huángqín

root of *Scutellaria baicalensis* and similar species (skullcap)
ALTERNATE NAME: *fǔcháng* "rotting intestines"
bitter flavor, balanced, non-toxic

Treats all sorts of heat, jaundice, intestinal afflux, and diarrhea; drives out water; moves down blood block; and [treats] malign sores, flat-abscesses and erosion, and fire sores. Grows in river valleys.

石龍芮

味苦，平，無毒

治風寒濕痹、心腹邪氣，利關節，止煩滿。久服輕身，明目，不老。生川澤石邊。

---

shílóngruì

whole plant of *Ranunculus sceleratus*
(cursed crowfoot/buttercup)
bitter flavor, balanced, non-toxic

Treats wind-, cold-, and damp-related *Bì* Impediment and evil qì in the heart and abdomen; disinhibits the joints; and stops vexation and fullness. Consumed over a long time, it lightens the body, brightens the eyes, and staves off aging. Grows in rivers and marshes on the side of rocks.

茅根

一名蘭根，一名茹根
味甘，寒，無毒

治勞傷、虛羸，補中益氣，除瘀血、血閉、寒熱，利小便。其苗，主下水。生山谷、田野。

---

máogēn

rhizome of *Imperata cylindrica* (cotton grass)
ALTERNATE NAMES: *lángén* "orchid root,"
rǔgēn "madder root"[8]
sweet flavor, cold, non-toxic

Treats taxation damage and vacuity emaciation; supplements the center and boosts qì; gets rid of static blood, blood block, and cold and heat; disinhibits urination. The shoots are indicated for moving down water. Grows in mountain valleys and open fields.

紫菀

一名青菀
味苦,溫,無毒

治欬逆上氣、胸中寒熱結氣,去蠱毒、痿厥,安五臟。生山谷。

---

zǐwǎn

"purple aster"
root and rhizome of *Aster tataricus* (Tartarian aster)
ALTERNATE NAME: qīngwǎn "green-blue aster"
bitter flavor, warm, non-toxic

Treats counterflow cough with ascent of qì, and cold and heat binding qì inside the chest; gets rid of *Gǔ* Toxin and wilting reversal; and calms the five *zàng* organs. Grows in mountain valleys.

紫草

一名紫丹,一名紫芙
味苦,寒,無毒

治心腹邪氣、五疸,補中益氣,利九竅,通水道。生山谷。

---

zǐcǎo

"purple grass"
root of *Lithospermum erythrorhizon* (purple gromwell)
ALTERNATE NAMES: *zǐdān* "purple cinnabar,"
zǐǎo "purple thistle"
bitter flavor, cold, non-toxic

Treats evil qì in the heart and abdomen and the five kinds of jaundice; supplements the center and boosts qì; disinhibits the Nine Orifices; and unclogs the waterways. Grows in mountain valleys.

茜根

味苦,寒,無毒

治寒濕風痹、黃疸,補中。生川谷。

qiàngēn

root of *Rubia cordifolia* (madder)
bitter flavor, cold, non-toxic

Treats cold-, damp-, and wind-related *Bì* Impediment and jaundice; and supplements the center. Grows in river valleys.

白鮮

味苦,寒,無毒

治頭風,黃疸,欬逆,淋瀝,女子陰中腫痛,濕痹,死肌不可屈伸、起止、行步。生川谷。

---

báixiān

"white renewal"
root bark of *Dictamnus dasycarpus* (dictamnus)
bitter, cold, non-toxic

Treats head wind; jaundice; counterflow cough; strangury and dribbling; women's swelling and pain inside the genitals; damp-related *Bì* Impediment; and dead flesh with inability to bend and stretch, to stand up and to rest, and to walk. Grows in river valleys.

酸漿

一名醋漿
味酸,平,無毒

治熱、煩滿,定志,益氣,利水道。產難,吞其實立產。生川澤及人家田園中。

---

suānjiāng

"sour liquid"
whole plant of *Physalis alkekengi* (Chinese lantern)
ALTERNATE NAME: *cùjiāng* "vinegar sauce"
sour flavor, balanced, non-toxic

Treats heat and vexation and fullness; settles the will; boosts qì; and disinhibits the waterways. For difficulties in childbirth, swallowing the fruit immediately induces the birth. Grows in rivers and marshes as well as in people's fields and gardens.

紫參

一名牡蒙
味苦,寒,無毒

治心腹積聚、寒熱邪氣,通九竅,利大小便,治牛病。生川谷。

zǐshēn

"purple *shēn*"
whole plant of *Salvia chinensis* (Chinese sage) or
Rubia yunnanensis (Yunnan madder)[9]
ALTERNATE NAME: *mǔméng* "bull dodder"
bitter flavor, cold, non-toxic

Treats accumulations and gatherings in the heart and abdomen and the evil qì of cold and heat; unclogs the Nine Orifices; disinhibits defecation and urination; and treats cattle disease. Grows in river valleys.

藁本

一名鬼卿,一名地新。
味辛,溫,無毒。

治婦人疝瘕、陰中寒腫痛、腹中急,除風頭痛,長肌膚,悅顏色。生山谷。

---

gǎoběn

rhizome and root of *Ligusticum sinense, jeholense,*
or *tenuissimum* (gaoben lovage)
ALTERNATE NAMES: *guǐqīng* "demon steward,"
dìxīn "native/earth new"
acrid flavor, warm, non-toxic

Treats women's *shàn*-type ("mounding") conglomerations, cold-related swelling and pain inside the genitals, and tension inside the abdomen; gets rid of wind head pain; makes the skin and flesh grow; and makes the complexion pleasant. Grows in mountain valleys.

狗脊

一名百枝
味苦，平，無毒

治腰背強，關機緩急，周痹，寒濕膝痛，頗利老人。生川谷。

---

gǒujǐ

"dog spine"
rhizome of *Cibotium barometz* (tree fern)
ALTERNATE NAME: *bǎizhī* "hundred branches"
bitter flavor, balanced, non-toxic

Treats rigidity in the lumbus and back, slackening and tensing in the barrier mechanisms,[10] pervasive *Bì* Impediment, and cold- and damp-related knee pain, and is particularly advantageous for older people. Grows in river valleys.

萆薢

味苦,平,無毒

治腰背痛,強骨節,風寒濕周痹,惡瘡不瘳,熱氣。生山谷。

---

bìxiè

rhizome of *Dioscorea hypoglauca, collettii, tokoro,*
or *gracillima* (fish poison yam)
bitter flavor, balanced, non-toxic

Treats pain in the lumbus and back; strengthens the bones and joints; [and treats] wind-, cold-, and damp-related pervasive *Bì* Impediment, malign sores that fail to heal, and heat qì. Grows in mountain valleys.

白兔藿

一名白葛
味苦,平,無毒

治蛇、虺、蜂、蠆、猘狗、菜、肉、蠱毒,鬼疰。生山谷。

---

báitùhuò

"white hare pulse"[11]
ALTERNATE NAME: *báigé* "white kudzu"
bitter flavor, balanced, non-toxic

Treats poisoning from snakes, vipers, wasps, scorpions, rabid dogs, vegetables and meat, and *Gǔ* Toxin as well as ghost infixation. Grows in mountain valleys.

營實

一名墻薇，一名墻麻，一名牛棘
味酸，溫，無毒

治癰疽、惡瘡、結肉趺筋、敗瘡、熱氣、陰蝕不瘳，利關節。 生川谷。

---

yíngshí

"provisioning fruit"
fruit of *Rosa multiflora* (multiflora rose)
ALTERNATE NAMES: *qiángwēi* "wall vetch,"
qiángmá "wall hemp," *niújí* "cow brambles"
sour flavor, warm, non-toxic

Treats welling- and flat-abscesses, malign sores, tumorous flesh and protruding sinews, putrefying wounds, heat qì, and genital erosion that fails to heal; and disinhibits the joints. Grows in river valleys.

薇銜

一名麋銜
味苦,平,無毒

治風濕痺,歷節痛,驚癇,吐舌,悸氣,賊風,鼠瘻,癰腫。生川澤。

---

wēixián

whole plant of *Pyrola rotundifolia*
(round-leaved wintergreen)
ALTERNATE NAME: *míxián* "elaphure snaffle"
bitter flavor, balanced, non-toxic

Treats wind- and damp-related *Bì* Impediment, joint-running pain, fright Seizures, protruding tongue, palpitation qì, Bandit Wind, Rat Fistulas, and swollen welling-abscesses. Grows in rivers and marshes.

水萍

一名水華
味辛,寒,無毒

治暴熱身癢,下水氣,勝酒,長須髮,止消渴。久服輕身。生池澤水上。

---

shuǐpíng

whole plant of *Spirodela polyrhiza* (common duckweed)
ALTERNATE NAME: *shuǐhuá* "water bloom"
acrid flavor, cold, non-toxic

Treats sudden heat with generalized itching, moves water qì down, overcomes liquor, makes the hair on the face and head grow, stops dispersion-thirst. Consumed over a long time, it lightens the body. Grows in lakes and marshes on top of the water.

王瓜

一名土瓜
味苦，寒，無毒

治消渴、內痺、瘀血、月閉、寒熱、酸疼，益氣，愈聾。生平澤田野及人家垣墻間。

---

wángguā

"king gourd"
fruit of *Trichosanthes cucumerina* (snake gourd)
ALTERNATE NAME: *tǔguā* "native gourd"
bitter flavor, cold, non-toxic

Treats dispersion thirst, internal *Bì* Impediment, static blood, menstrual block, cold and heat, and soreness; boosts qì; and cures deafness. Grows in marshy flatlands and wild fields, as well as between the walls of people's courtyards.

地榆

味苦，微寒，無毒

治婦人乳痓痛、七傷、帶下十二病，止痛，除惡肉，止汗氣，消酒，明目，治金瘡。生山谷。

---

dìyú

"native elm"
root of *Sanguisorba officinalis* (great burnet)
bitter flavor, slightly cold, non-toxic

Treats women's spasms and pain in the breast, the Seven Damages, and the Twelve Diseases Below the Girdle; stops pain; gets rid of malign flesh; stops sweat qì,[12] disperses liquor, brightens the eyes, and treats incised wounds. Grows in mountain valleys.

海藻

一名落首
味苦，寒，無毒

治癭瘤氣、頸下核，破散結氣、癰腫、癥瘕堅氣，腹中上下鳴，下十二水腫。生東海池澤。

---

hǎizǎo

whole plant of *Sargassum fusiforme* or *pallidum* (hijiki)
ALTERNATE NAME: *luòshǒu* "dropping head"
bitter flavor, cold, non-toxic

Treats the qì of goiters and tumors of the neck and nodes underneath the neck; breaks up and scatters bound qì, swollen welling-abscesses, and concretions, accumulations, and firmed qì; [treats] rumbling inside and above and below the abdomen; and moves down the twelve [kinds of] water swelling. Grows in the East China Sea and in lakes and marshes.

澤蘭

一名虎蘭，一名龍棗
味苦，微溫，無毒

治乳婦衄血，中風餘疾，大腹水腫，身面四肢浮腫，骨節中水，金瘡，癰腫瘡膿。生諸大澤旁。

---

zélán

"marsh orchid"
foliage and stalk of *Lycopus lucidus* (bugleweed)
ALTERNATE NAMES: *hǔlán* "tiger orchid,"
lóngzǎo "dragon jujube"
bitter flavor, slightly warm, non-toxic

Treats Spontaneous Bleeding in breastfeeding mothers, residual diseases after wind strike, water swelling in the greater abdomen, puffy swelling in the body, face, and four limbs, water inside the bones and joints, incised wounds, swollen welling-abscesses and suppurating sores. Grows alongside all sorts of large swamps.

防己

一名解離
味辛,平,無毒

治風寒、溫瘧、熱氣、諸癇,除邪,利大小便。生川谷。

---

fángjǐ

"fend off self"
root of *Aristolochia fangshi* or *heterophylla*[13] (birthwort)
ALTERNATE NAME: *jiělí* "resolve and separate"
acrid flavor, balanced, non-toxic

Treats wind and cold, warm malaria, heat qì, and all sorts of Seizures; expels evil; and disinhibits defecation and urination. Grows in river valleys.

牡丹

一名鹿韭，一名鼠姑
味辛，寒，無毒

治寒熱、中風、瘈瘲、痙、驚癇邪氣，除癥堅、瘀血留舍腸胃，安五藏，療癰瘡。生山谷。

---

mǔdān

"male cinnabar"
bark of the root of *Paeonia suffruticosa* (moutan)
ALTERNATE NAMES: *lùjiǔ* "deer chive," *shǔgū* "rat maiden"
acrid flavor, cold, non-toxic

Treats the evil qì of cold and heat, wind strike, convulsions, tetany, and fright Seizures; gets rid of concretions and firmness and static blood lodging in the intestines and stomach; calms the five *zàng* organs; and cures welling-abscesses. Grows in mountain valleys.

款冬花

一名橐吾，一名顆東，一名虎須，一名菟奚
味辛，溫，無毒

治欬逆上氣，善喘，喉痹，諸驚癇，寒熱邪氣。生山谷及水旁。

---

kuǎndōnghuā

flower of *Tussilago farfara* (coltsfoot)
ALTERNATE NAMES: *tuówú* "bellows defender,"
kēdòng "granule rainstorm," *hǔxū* "tiger's whiskers,"
túxī "dodder slave"
acrid flavor, warm, non-toxic

Treats counterflow cough with ascent of qì, tendency to panting, *Bì* Impediment in the throat, all sorts of fright Seizures, and the evil qì of cold and heat. Grows in mountain valleys and alongside water.

石韋

味苦,平,無毒

治勞熱邪氣、五癃、閉不通,利小便水道。生山谷石上。

---

shíwéi

"stone leather"
foliage of *Pyrrosia lingua* and other species (pyrrosia fern)
bitter flavor, balanced, non-toxic

Treats the evil qì of taxation heat, the five [kinds of] dribbling urinary stoppage, and [urinary] blockage and clog; and disinhibits the urine and waterways. Grows in mountain valleys on top of rocks.

馬先蒿

一名馬屎蒿
味苦，平，無毒

治寒熱，鬼疰，中風，濕痹，女子帶下病、無子。生川澤。

---

mǎxiānhāo

"horse prior wormwood"
whole plant of *Pedicularis resupinata* (inverted lousewort)
ALTERNATE NAME: *mǎshǐhāo* "horse dung wormwood"
bitter flavor, balanced, non-toxic

Treats cold and heat, ghost infixation, wind strike, damp-related *Bì* Impediment, and women's disorders of vaginal discharge and infertility. Grows in rivers and marshes.

女菀

味辛,溫,無毒

治風寒灑灑,霍亂,泄利,腸鳴上下無常處,驚癇,寒熱百疾。生川谷或山陽。

---

nǚwǎn

"female aster"
whole plant or roots of *Aster fastigiatus*
acrid flavor, warm, non-toxic

Treats wind and cold with shivering, Sudden Turmoil, diarrhea, intestinal rumbling that ascends and descends with no constant location, fright Seizures, and the hundred illnesses of cold and heat. Grows in river valleys or on the south-facing side of mountains.

王孫

吳名白功艸,楚名王孫,齊名長孫
味苦,平,無毒

治五臟邪氣,寒濕痹,四肢疼酸,膝冷痛。生川谷及城郭垣下。

---

wángsūn

"king's descendant"
rhizome of *Paris tetraphylla* (four-leaved paris)
ALTERNATE NAMES: In Wú, *báigōngcǎo* "white merit herb,"
in Chǔ, *wángsūn* "royal descendant,"
in Qí, *zhǎngsūn* "eldest son's eldest son"
bitter flavor, balanced, non-toxic

Treats evil qì in the five *zàng* organs, cold- and damp-related *Bì* Impediment, soreness in the four limbs, and cold pain in the knees. Grows in river valleys and below city walls and ramparts.

雲實

味辛,溫,無毒

治泄利、腸澼,殺蟲、蠱毒,去邪惡、結氣,止痛,除寒熱。華,主見鬼精物,多食令人狂走。久服輕身,通神明。生川谷。

---

yúnshí

"cloud seed"

seed of *Caesalpinia sepiaria* (cat's claw/Mysore thorn)

acrid flavor, warm, non-toxic

Treats diarrhea and intestinal afflux; kills worms and Gǔ Toxin; gets rid of evil malignity and bound qì; stops pain; and gets rid of cold and heat. The flowers are indicated for seeing ghosts ad spectral entities, and make a person run around manically if eaten in large quantities. Consumed over a long time, it lightens the body and facilitates the breakthrough of spirit illumination. Grows in river valleys.

爵床

味鹹,寒,無毒

治腰脊痛不得著床、俛仰艱難,除熱。可作浴湯。生川谷及田野。

---

juéchuáng

"sparrow bed"

whole plant of *Rostellularia procumbens*[14] (water willow)

salty flavor, cold, non-toxic

Treats pain in the lumbus and spine that prevents the patient from lying flat on the bed, and bending forward and backward only with great difficulty; and gets rid of heat. Can be prepared as a medicinal bath. Grows in river valleys and open fields.

黃耆

一名戴糝
味甘，微溫，無毒

治癰疽、久敗瘡，排膿止痛，大風癩疾、五痔、鼠瘻，補虛，小兒百病。生山谷。

huángqí

"yellow attainment"
root of *Astragalus membranaceus, mongholicus*,
and other species (vetch)
ALTERNATE NAME: *dàishēn*
sweet flavor, slightly warm, non-toxic

Treats welling- and flat-abscesses and chronic putrefying sores; pushes out pus and stops pain; [treats] great wind *lài* leprosy, the five [kinds of] Hemorrhoids, and Rat Fistulas; supplements emptiness; and [treats] the hundred diseases of small children. Grows in mountain valleys.

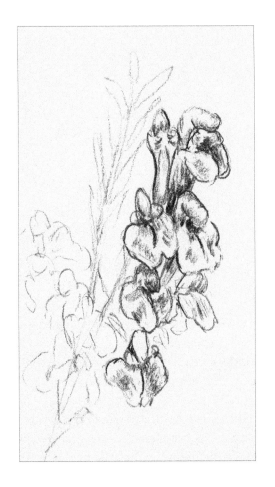

Sketch 12 - *huángqí*

黃連

一名王連
味苦,寒,無毒

治熱氣、目痛、眥傷、泣出,明目,腸澼、腹痛、下利、婦人陰中腫痛。久服令人不忘。生川谷。

---

huánglián

"yellow connection"
rhizome of *Coptis chinensis, deltoidea,*
and other species (coptis)
ALTERNATE NAME: *wánglián* "royal connection"
bitter flavor, cold, non-toxic

Treats heat qì, eye pain, damage to the corner of the eyes, and tearing; brightens the eyes; and [treats] intestinal afflux, abdominal pain, diarrhea, and women's swelling and pain inside the genitals. Consumed over a long time, it staves off forgetfulness. Grows in river valleys.

五味子

一名會及
味酸,溫,無毒

主益氣、欬逆上氣、勞傷羸瘦,補不足,強陰,益男子精。生山谷。

---

wǔwèizǐ

"five flavor seed"
fruit of *Schisandra chinensis*
ALTERNATE NAME: *huìjí* "gather to reach"
sour flavor, warm, non-toxic

Indicated for boosting qì, counterflow cough with ascent of qì, and taxation damage with gauntness; supplementing insufficiency; strengthening yīn; and boosting *jīng* essence in men. Grows in mountain valleys.

沙參

一名知母
味苦,微寒,無毒

治血積、驚氣,除寒熱,補中,益肺氣。久服利人。生川谷。

---

shāshēn

"sand *shēn*"
root of *Adenophora tetraphylla* and similar species (ladybell)
ALTERNATE NAME: *zhīmǔ* "mother of knowing"
bitter flavor, slightly cold, non-toxic

Treats blood accumulations and fright qì, gets rid of cold and heat, supplements the center, and boosts lung qì. Consumed over a long time, it is beneficial. Grows in river valleys.

桔梗

味辛,微溫,有小毒

治胸脅痛如刀刺,腹滿,腸鳴幽幽,驚恐悸氣。生山谷。

---

jiégěng

root of *Platycodon grandiflorum* (balloon flower)
acrid flavor, slightly warm, slightly toxic

Treats pain in the chest and rib-sides as if being stabbed with a knife, abdominal fullness, deep rumbling in the intestines, and the qì of fright and fear palpitations. Grows in mountain valleys.

莨菪子

一名橫唐
味苦,寒,有毒

治齒痛,出蟲,肉痹拘急,使人健行、見鬼。多食令人狂走。久服輕身,走及奔馬,強志,益力,通神。生海濱、川谷。

làngdàngzǐ

seed of *Hyoscyamus niger* (henbane)
ALTERNATE NAME: *héngtáng* "transverse boasting"
bitter flavor, cold, toxic

Treats tooth pain, makes worms leave, [treats] *Bì* Impediment in the flesh with hypertonicity, and makes you walk with vigor and see ghosts. If eaten in large quantities, it causes you to run around manically. Consumed over a long time, it lightens the body, makes you run as fast as a galloping horse, strengthens the will, boosts strength, and facilitates the breakthrough of spirit [illumination]. Grows on the shores of large bodies of water and in river valleys.

陸英

味苦,寒,無毒

治骨間諸痺,四肢拘攣、疼酸,膝寒痛,陰痿,短氣不足,腳腫。生川谷。

---

lùyīng

"dryland bloom"
fruit of *Sambucus javanica* (Chinese elder)
bitter flavor, cold, non-toxic

Treats all sorts of *Bì* Impediment in the space of the bones, hypertonicity and soreness in the four limbs, cold pain in the knees, Yīn Wilt, shortness of breath and insufficiency, and swelling in the feet. Grows in river valleys.

姑活

一名冬葵子
味甘,溫,無毒

治大風,邪氣,濕痹寒痛。久服輕身,益壽,耐老。

---

gūhuó[15]

"maiden life"
ALTERNATE NAME: *dōngkuízǐ* "winter mallow seed"
sweet flavor, warm, non-toxic

Treats great wind, evil qì, and damp-related *Bì* Impediment with cold and pain. Consumed over a long time, it lightens the body, boosts longevity, and makes aging tolerable.

屈草

味苦,微寒,無毒

治胸脅下痛,邪氣,腹閒寒熱,陰痹。久服輕身,益氣,耐老。生川澤。

---

qūcǎo[16]

"curled grass"
bitter flavor, slightly cold, non-toxic

Treats pain below the chest and rib-sides, evil qì, cold and heat in the abdominal region, and yīn-type *Bì* Impediment. Consumed over a long time, it lightens the body, boosts qì, and makes aging tolerable. Grows in rivers and marshes.

別羈

味苦，微溫，無毒

治風寒濕痹，身重，四肢疼酸，寒邪，歷節痛。生川谷。

---

biéjī[17]

"separate bridle"
bitter flavor, slightly warm, non-toxic

Treats wind-, cold-, and damp-related *Bì* Impediment, generalized heaviness, soreness in the four limbs, cold evil, and joint-running pain. Grows in river valleys.

翹根

味甘,寒,有小毒

治下熱氣,益陰精,令人面悅好,明目。久服輕身,耐老。生平澤。

---

qiáogēn[18]

"upward-arching root"
sweet flavor, cold, slightly toxic

Treats heat qì by moving it downward, boosts yīn [and] essence,[19] makes your face pleasing and beautiful, and brightens the eyes. Consumed over a long time, it lightens the body and makes aging tolerable. Grows in marshy flatlands.

萱草

一名忘憂，一名宜男，一名歧女
味甘，平，無毒

主安五臟，利心志，令人好歡樂無憂，輕身，明目。

---

xuāncǎo

root of *Hemerocallis vulva*[20] (orange day-lily)
ALTERNATE NAMES: *wàngyōu* "forget your sorrows,"
yínán "suited to male," *qínǚ* "diverging female"
sweet flavor, balanced, non-toxic

Indicated for calming the five *zàng* organs; disinhibiting the heart and will; making you beautiful, joyful, and worry-free; lightening the body; and brightening the eyes.

中藥

Middle Medicinals

木部

Trees

梔子

一名木丹
味苦,寒,無毒

治五內邪氣,胃中熱氣,面赤,酒皰皶鼻,白癩,赤癩,瘡瘍。生川谷。

---

zhīzǐ

fruit of *Gardenia jasminoides* (cape jasmine)
ALTERNATE NAME: *mùdān* "tree peony"
bitter flavor, cold, non-toxic

Treats the five [kinds of] internal evil qì, heat qì inside the stomach, redness of the face, liquor blisters and drunkard's nose, White *Lài* Leprosy, red *lài* leprosy, and skin conditions [in general]. Grows in river valleys.

竹葉

味苦,平,無毒

治欬逆上氣、溢筋急、惡瘍,殺小蟲。根,作湯,益氣,止渴,補虛,下氣。汁,治風痓。實,通神明,輕身,益氣。

---

zhúyè

"bamboo leaves"
foliage of Phyllostachys nigra and related species
(bamboo)
bitter flavor, balanced, non-toxic

Treats counterflow cough with ascent of qì, spilling sinew tension, and malign sores; and kills small worms. The roots, prepared as a decoction, boost qì, stop thirst, supplement emptiness, and move down qì. The juice treats wind tetany. The seed facilitates the breakthrough of spirit illumination, lightens the body, and boosts qì.

檗木

一名檀桓
味苦,寒,無毒

治五臟腸胃中結熱、黃疸、腸痔,止泄利,女下漏下赤白、陰傷、蝕瘡。生山谷。

bòmù

bark of *Phellodendron amurense* (cork tree bark)
ALTERNATE NAME: *tánhuán* "sandalwood pillar"
bitter flavor, cold, non-toxic

Treats bound heat inside the five *zàng* organs and the intestines and stomach, jaundice, and intestinal Hemorrhoids; stops diarrhea; and [treats] women's vaginal leaking and red and white discharge, damage to the genitals, and erosion sores. Grows in mountain valleys.

吳茱萸

一名藙
味辛，溫，有小毒

主溫中，下氣，止痛，欬逆，寒熱，除濕，血痹，逐風邪，開腠理。根，溫，殺三蟲。久服輕身。生川谷。

wúzhūyú

unripe fruit of *Tetradium ruticarpum* (evodia)
ALTERNATE NAME: *yì*[21]
acrid flavor, warm, slightly toxic

Indicated for warming the center, moving down qì, stopping pain, counterflow cough, cold and heat, getting rid of dampness and [treating] blood *Bì* Impediment, driving out wind evil, and opening up the interstices. The roots are warm and kill the Three Worms. Consumed over a long time, it lightens the body. Grows in river valleys.

桑根白皮

味甘,寒,無毒

治傷中、五勞、六極、羸瘦、崩中、脈絕,補虛,益氣。葉,主除寒熱,出汗。桑耳,平。黑者,治女子漏下赤白汁,血病,癥瘕積聚,陰痛,陰陽寒熱,無子。五木耳,一名檽,益氣,不飢,輕身,強志。生山谷。

---

sānggēnbáipí

"white bark of mulberry root"
bark of the root of *Morus alba*
sweet flavor, cold, non-toxic

Treats damage to the center, the Five Taxations and Six Extremes, gauntness, [vaginal] flooding from the center, and a severed pulse; supplements emptiness; and boosts qì. The leaves are indicated for getting rid of cold and heat and for ousting sweat. Mulberry wood ear (*Auricularia auricula*) is balanced. The black [variety] treats women's vaginal spotting with red and white liquid; blood disease; concretions, conglomerations, accumulations, and gatherings; pain in the genitals; genital sores[22] with cold and heat; and infertility. Fivefold wood ear,[23] also called *ruǎn*, boosts qì, staves off aging, lightens the body, and strengthens the will. Grows in mountain valleys.

蕪荑

一名無姑
味辛,平,無毒

治五內邪氣,散皮膚骨節中淫淫行毒,去三蟲,化食,逐寸白,散腹中嗢嗢喘息。生川谷。

wúyí

processed fruit of *Ulmus macrocarpa* (elm preparation)
ALTERNATE NAME: *wúgū*
acrid flavor, balanced, non-toxic

Treats the five [kinds of] internal evil qì; scatters wantonly spreading toxin in the skin, bones, and joints; gets rid off the Three Worms; transforms food; drives out Inch Whiteworm;[24] and scatters gurgling sounds inside the abdomen with panting. Grows in river valleys.

枳實

味苦，寒，無毒

治大風在皮膚中、如麻豆苦癢，除寒熱結，止利，長肌肉，利五臟，益氣，輕身。生川澤。

---

zhǐshí

unripe fruit of *Poncirus trifoliata* or *Citrus aurantium* or *Citrus x wilsonii* (bitter orange)
bitter flavor, cold, non-toxic

Treats great wind located inside the skin and a feeling like measles and smallpox with severe itching; gets rid of wind and heat binds; stops disinhibited [defecation]; grows flesh; disinhibits the five *zàng* organs; boosts qì; and lightens the body. Grows in rivers and marshes.

厚朴

味苦,溫,無毒

治中風、傷寒、頭痛、寒熱、驚悸氣、血痹、死肌,去三蟲。生山谷。

---

hòupò

bark of *Magnolia officinalis* or *biloba* (official magnolia bark)
bitter flavor, warm, non-toxic

Treats wind strike, cold damage, headache, cold and heat, fright palpitation qì, blood *Bì* Impediment, and dead flesh; and gets rid of the Three Worms. Grows in mountain valleys.

秦皮

味苦,微寒,無毒

治風寒濕痺、灑灑寒氣,除熱、目中青翳白膜。久服頭不白,輕身。生川谷。

---

qínpí

bark of the trunk of *Fraxinus rhynchophylla* and
related species (ash bark)
bitter flavor, slightly cold, non-toxic

Treats wind-, cold- and damp-related *Bì* Impediment and shivering with cold qì; and gets rid of heat and green-blue screens and white films over the middle of the eyes. Consumed for a long time, it staves off whitening of the [hair on the] head and lightens the body. Grows in river valleys.

秦椒

味辛,溫,有毒

治風邪氣,溫中,除寒痹,堅齒,長髮,明目。久服輕身,好顏色,耐老,增年,通神。生川谷。

---

qínjiāo

"Shenxi pepper"
seed capsule of *Zanthoxylum bungeanum*
acrid flavor, warm, toxic

Treats wind evil qì, warms the center, gets rid of cold-related *Bì* Impediment, makes the teeth firm, grows the hair on the head, and brightens the eyes. Consumed over a long period of time, it lightens the body, makes the complexion beautiful, allows you to withstand aging, increases the years, and facilitates the breakthrough of spirit [illumination]. Grows in river valleys.

山茱萸

一名蜀棗
味酸,平,無毒

治心下邪氣、寒熱,溫中,逐寒濕痹,去三蟲。久服輕身。生山谷。

---

shānzhūyú

"mountain *zhūyú*"
fruit of *Cornus officinalis* (dogwood)
ALTERNATE NAME: *shǔzǎo* "Western Sìchuān jujube"
sour flavor, balanced, non-toxic

Treats evil qì below the heart and cold and heat; warms the center; drives out cold- and damp-related *Bì* Impediment; and gets rid of the Three Worms. Consumed over a long period of time, it lightens the body. Grows in mountain valleys.

紫葳

一名芙華,一名陵苕
味酸,微寒,無毒

治婦人產乳餘疾、崩中、癥瘕、血閉、寒熱、羸瘦,養胎。生西海川谷及山陽。

---

zǐwēi

"purple lushness"
flower of *Campsis grandiflora* (trumpet creeper)
ALTERNATE NAMES: *ǎohuá* "ǎo flower," *língtiáo* [25]
sour flavor, slightly cold, non-toxic

Treats women's residual diseases after childbearing and breastfeeding, Center Flooding, concretions and conglomerations, blood block, cold and heat, and gauntness; and nurtures the fetus. Grows in the river valleys of the far west and on the south-facing sides of mountains.

豬苓

一名豭豬屎
味甘,平,無毒

治痎瘧,解毒、蠱疰、不祥,利水道。久服輕身,耐老。生山谷。

---

zhūlíng

"pig truffle"
fruiting body of *Polyporus umbellata* (umbrella polypore)
ALTERNATE NAME: *jiāzhūshǐ* "boar manure"
sweet flavor, balanced, non-toxic

Treats malaria, resolves toxins, *gǔ* infixation, and bad luck; and disinhibits the waterways. Consumed over a long period of time, it lightens the body and allows you to withstand aging. Grows in mountain valleys.

白棘

一名棘鍼
味辛,寒,無毒

治心腹痛、癰腫潰膿,止痛。生川谷。

---

báijí

"white jujube/thorn"
thorns of *Ziziphus jujuba* (jujube thorns)
ALTERNATE NAME: *jízhēn* "jujube needle"
acrid flavor, cold, non-toxic

Treats heart and abdominal pain and swollen ulcerating welling-abscesses; and stops pain. Grows in river valleys.

龍眼

一名益智
味甘,平,無毒

治五臟邪氣,安志,厭食。久服強魂魄,聰明,輕身,不老,通神明。生南海山谷。

---

lóngyǎn

"dragon eye"
fruit of *Dimocarpus longan* (longan)
ALTERNATE NAME: *yìzhì* "wisdom-booster"
sweet flavor, balanced, non-toxic

Treats evil *qì* in the five *zàng* organs, calms the will, and satisfies the appetite. Consumed over a long time, it strengthens the *hún* and *pò* souls, makes you sharp and bright, lightens the body, staves off aging, and facilitates the breakthrough of spirit illumination. Grows in mountain valleys in the far south.

木蘭

一名林蘭
味苦，寒，無毒

治身大熱在皮膚中，去面熱、赤皰、酒皶，惡風，癲疾，陰下癢濕。明耳目。生川谷。

---

mùlán

"wood orchid"
bark of *Magnolia liliflora* (lily magnolia)
ALTERNATE NAME: *línlán* "forest orchid"
bitter flavor, cold, non-toxic

Treats great heat inside the skin all over the body; gets rid of heat in the face, red blisters, and a drunkard's nose; and treats malign wind, Epilepsy,[26] and itching and dampness below the genitals. Brightens the ears and eyes. Grows in river valleys.

桑上寄生

一名寄屑,一名寓木,一名宛童。
味苦,平,無毒。

治腰痛、小兒背強、癰腫,安胎,充肌膚,堅髮齒,長鬚眉。其實,明目,輕身,通神。生川谷桑樹上。

---

sāngshàngjìshēng

"mulberry parasite"

branches and foliage of *Viscum coloratum* or *Loranthus parasiticus* and related species (mulberry mistletoe)

ALTERNATE NAMES: *jìxiè* "parasitic flakes,"
yùmù "tree sojourner," *wǎntóng* "supple youth"

bitter flavor, balanced, non-toxic

Treats lumbar pain, rigidity in the spine in small children, and swollen welling-abscess, calms the fetus, fills out the skin and flesh, makes the hair on the head and the teeth firm, and makes the beard and eyebrows grow. Its fruit brightens the eyes, lightens the body, and facilitates the breakthrough of spirit [illumination]. Grows in river valleys on mulberry trees.

柳花

一名柳絮
味苦,寒,無毒

治風水,黃疸,面熱黑。葉,治馬疥、痂瘡。實,主潰癰,逐膿血。生川澤。

liǔhuā

"willow flower"
flower of *Salix babylonica*
ALTERNATE NAME: *liúxù* "willow catkins"
bitter flavor, cold, non-toxic

Treats Wind Water,[27] jaundice, and heat and blackness in the face. The leaves treat Horse Scabies and mange. The fruits are indicated for rupturing welling-abscesses and driving out pus and blood. Grows in rivers and marshes.

衛矛

一名鬼箭
味苦,寒,無毒

治女子崩中下血、腹滿、汗出,除邪,殺鬼、毒、蠱注。生山谷。

---

wèimáo

"spear of protection"
branch or plumes of *Euonymus elatus* (winged spindle tree)
ALTERNATE NAME: *guǐjiàn* "demon arrow"
bitter flavor, cold, non-toxic

Treats women's Center Flooding and vaginal bleeding, abdominal fullness, and sweating; expels evils; and kills demons, toxins, and *gǔ* influx. Grows in mountain valleys.

合歡

一名蠲忿
味甘，平，無毒

主安五臟，和心志，令人歡無憂。久服輕身，明目，得所欲。生山谷。

---

héhuān

"conjoined rejoicing"
bark of *Albizzia julibrissin* [28] (silk tree)
ALTERNATE NAME: *juānfèn* "wrath-eliminator"
sweet flavor, balanced, non-toxic

Indicated for quieting the five *zàng* organs, harmonizing the heart and will, and making you joyous and free from worries. Consumed over a long time, it lightens the body, brightens the eyes, and gets you what you want. Grows in mountain valleys.

松蘿

一名女蘿
味苦,平,無毒

治瞋怒、邪氣,止虛汗、頭風,女子陰寒腫病。生川谷松樹上。

---

sōngluó

"pine vine"
whole plant of *Usnea longissima* (beard-lichen)
ALTERNATE NAME: *nǚluó* "female vine"
bitter flavor, balanced, non-toxic

Treats glaring fury and evil qì; stops emptiness sweat and head wind; and [treats] women's cold in the genitals and swelling disease. Grows in river valleys on pine trees.

乾漆

味辛,溫,無毒

治絕傷,補中,續筋骨,填髓腦,安五臟,五緩六急,風寒濕痹。生漆,去長蟲。久服輕身,耐老。生川谷。

gānqī

"dried lacquer"
dried sap of *Toxicodendron vernicifluum* (lacquer)
acrid flavor, warm, non-toxic

Treats damage from severance; supplements the center; reconnects sinews and bones; replenishes the marrow and brain; calms the five *zàng* organs; and [treats] the five slacknesses and six tightnesses and wind-, cold-, and damp-related *Bì* Impediment. The fresh sap gets rid of long worms. Consumed over a long time, it lightens the body and allows you to withstand aging. Grows in river valleys.

石南

一名鬼目
味辛,平,有毒

主養腎氣,內傷陰衰,利筋骨皮毛。實,殺蟲毒,破積聚,逐風痹。生山谷。

---

shínán

"stone south"

leaves of *Photinia serratifolia* (Taiwanese photinia)

ALTERNATE NAME: *guǐmù* "demon's eye"

acrid flavor, balanced, toxic

Indicated for nourishing kidney qì, [treating] internal damage [causing] debilitation of yīn, and disinhibiting the joints, bones, skin, and body hair. The fruits kill *Gǔ* Toxins, break gatherings and accumulations, and drive out wind-related *Bì* Impediment. Grows in mountain valleys.

蔓椒

一名豕椒
味苦,溫,無毒

治風寒濕痺歷節疼,除四肢厥氣、膝痛。生川谷及邱冢間。

---

mànjiāo[29]

"creeping prickly-ash"
root or foliage of *Zanthoxylum nitidum*
(shiny-leaf prickly-ash)
ALTERNATE NAME: *shǐjiāo* "pig prickly-ash"
bitter flavor, warm, non-toxic

Treats wind-, cold-, and damp-related *Bì* Impediment with joint-running pain and gets rid of reversal qì in the four limbs and knee pain. Grows in river valleys and around grave mounds.

欒華

味苦,寒,無毒

治目痛、淚出、傷眥,消目腫。生川谷。

---

luánhuá

flower of *Koelreuteria paniculata* (goldenrain)
bitter flavor, cold, non-toxic

Treats eye pain, tearing, and damage to the corners of the eyes, and disperses swelling of the eye. Grows in river valleys.

淮木

一名百歲城中木
味苦，平，無毒

治久欬上氣，傷中，虛羸，女子陰蝕、漏下赤白沃。生平澤。

---

huáimù[30]

"Huái Tree"
ALTERNATE NAME: *bǎisuìchéngzhōngmù*
"hundred-year city-center tree"
bitter flavor, balanced, non-toxic

Treats long-term coughing with qì ascent, damage to the center, vacuity and gauntness, and women's genital erosion, vaginal spotting, and red and white soaking. Grows in marshy flatlands.

中藥
MIDDLE MEDICINALS

穀部
FOOD CROPS

梅實

味酸,平,無毒

主下氣,除熱、煩滿,安心,止肢體痛,偏枯不仁,死肌,去青黑痣、惡疾,能益氣,不饑。生川谷。

méishí

fruit of *Prunus mume*
(fruit of the Japanese apricot, a.k.a. mume)[31]
sour flavor, balanced, non-toxic

Indicated for moving qì down; getting rid of heat and vexation with fullness; calming the heart; and stopping pain in the limbs and trunk; for hemilateral withering and numbness, and dead flesh; for getting rid of green-blue or black moles and malign conditions; and for being able to boost qì and staving off hunger. Grows in river valleys.

蓼實

味辛,溫,無毒

主明目,溫中,耐風寒,下水氣,面目浮腫,癰瘍。馬蓼,去腸中蛭蟲,輕身。生川澤。

---

liǎoshí

fruit of *Polygonum hydropiper* (knotweed)
acrid flavor, warm, non-toxic

Indicated for brightening the eyes, warming the center, allowing you to withstand wind and cold, moving down water qì, and for puffy swelling in the face and eyes and for welling-abscesses and open sores. *Mǎliǎo* (horse knotweed, *Polygonum persicaria*) gets rid of intestinal flukes and lightens the body. Grows in rivers and marshes.

蔥實

味辛,溫,無毒

主明目,補中不足。其莖,平,作湯,治傷寒、寒熱、出汗、中風、面目腫。薤,味辛,溫,無毒。治金瘡瘡敗,輕身,不飢,耐老。生平澤。

cōngshí

seed of *Allium fistulosum* (scallion)
acrid flavor, warm, non-toxic

Indicated for brightening the eyes and supplementing insufficiency in the center. The stalk is balanced and, when prepared as a decoction, treats cold damage, cold and heat, sweating, wind strike, and swelling in the face and eyes. The bulb is acrid in flavor, warm, and non-toxic. It treats incised wounds and wound putrefaction, lightens the body, staves off hunger, and allows you to withstand aging. Grows in marshy flatlands.

水蘇

一名芥蒩
味辛,微溫,無毒

主下氣,殺穀,除飲食,辟口臭,去毒,辟惡氣。久服通神明,輕身,耐老。生池澤。

---

shuǐsū

"water reviver"
whole plant of *Stachys baicalensis* (water betony)
ALTERNATE NAME: *jièjū* "mustard green fishwort"
acrid flavor, slightly warm, non-toxic

Indicated for bringing down the qì, killing grain,[32] expelling drink and food, warding off foul breath, getting rid of toxins, and warding off malign qì. Consumed over a long time, it facilitates the breakthrough of spirit illumination, lightens the body, and allows you to withstand aging. Grows in ponds and marshes.

瓜蒂

味苦,寒,有毒

治大水身面四肢浮腫,下水,殺蠱毒,欬逆上氣,及食諸果不消,病在胸腹中,皆吐下之。生平澤。

guādì

"gourd stalk"
peduncle of various species of *Cucumis*
bitter flavor, cold, toxic

Treats severe water [qì] with puffy swelling all over the body, in the face, and in the four limbs; moves water down; kills *Gǔ* Toxins; and [treats] counterflow cough with ascent of qì as well as failure to digest all sorts of fruits after eating them. In all cases of disease in the chest or abdomen, [*guādì* eliminates them by] vomiting them up or moving them down. Grows in marshy flatlands.

水蘄

一名水英
味甘,平,無毒

治女子赤沃,止血,養精,保血脈,益氣,令人肥健、嗜食。生南海池澤。

---

shuǐqín

"water-dropwort"
whole plant of *Oenanthe javanica* (Chinese celery)
ALTERNATE NAME: *shuǐyīng* "water bloom"
sweet flavor, balanced, non-toxic

Treats women's red [vaginal] soaking, stops bleeding, nourishes the essence, safeguards the flow of blood in the vessels, boosts qì, makes you plump and healthy, and causes you to crave food. Grows in ponds and marshes in the far south.

粟米

味鹹,微寒,無毒

主養腎氣,去胃脾中熱,益氣。陳粟,味苦,寒,無毒。主胃熱、消渴,利小便。

---

sùmǐ

seed of *Setaria italica* (foxtail millet)
salty flavor, slightly cold, non-toxic

Indicated for nurturing kidney qì, getting rid of heat inside the stomach and spleen, and boosting qì. Aged millet is bitter in flavor, cold, and non-toxic. It is indicated for stomach heat and dispersion thirst, and disinhibits urination.

黍米

味甘,溫,無毒

主益氣補中,多熱令人煩。丹黍米,味苦,微溫。主欬逆、霍亂,止泄,除熱,止煩渴。

---

shǔmǐ

seed of *Panicum miliaceum* (broomcorn millet)
sweet flavor, warm, non-toxic

Indicated for boosting qì and supplementing the center and for copious heat that is causing vexation.[33] Cinnabar broomcorn millet[34] is bitter in flavor and slightly warm. It is in charge of counterflow cough and Sudden Turmoil, stops diarrhea, gets rid of heat, and stops vexation with thirst.

麻蕡

一名麻勃
味辛,平,有毒

治五勞七傷,利五臟,下血,寒氣。多食令人見鬼狂走。久服通神明,輕身。生川谷。麻子,味甘,平,無毒。主補中益氣。久服肥健,不老。

---

máfén

achene[35] of *Cannabis sativa* (hemp seed)
ALTERNATE NAME: *mábó* hemp flowers
acrid flavor, balanced, toxic

Treats the five taxations and Seven Damages, disinhibits the five *zàng* organs, moves the blood down, and [treats] cold qì. Eaten in large quantities, it causes you to see ghosts and run around manically. Consumed over a long time, it facilitates the breakthrough of spirit illumination and lightens the body. Grows in river valleys. The [inner] seed of hemp is sweet in flavor, balanced, and non-toxic. It is indicated for supplementing the center and boosting qì. Consumed over a long time, it makes you plump and strong and staves off aging.

中藥
Middle Medicinals

石部
Rocks

石硫黃

味酸,溫,有毒

治婦人陰蝕、疽、痔、惡瘡,堅筋骨,除頭禿,能化金、銀、銅、鐵、奇物。青白色,主益肝,明目。生東海、山谷中。

---

shíliúhuáng

sulfur

sour flavor, warm, toxic

Treats women's genital erosion, flat-abscesses, Hemorrhoids, and malign sores; makes the sinews and bones firm; gets rid of baldness; and is able to transform gold, silver, copper, iron, and strange substances. [Sulfur compounds] that are green-blue or white in color are indicated for boosting the liver and brightening the eyes. Grows in mountain valleys by the East China Sea.[36]

石膏

味辛,微寒,無毒

治中風寒熱、心下逆氣、驚喘、口乾、舌焦、不能息、腹中堅痛,除邪鬼,產乳,金瘡。生山谷。

---

shígāo

"stone lard"

gypsum

acrid flavor, slightly cold, non-toxic

Treats wind strike with cold and heat, counterflow qì below the heart, fright with panting, dry mouth and parched tongue, inability to breathe, and firmness and pain inside the abdomen; expels evil and demons; and [treats problems associated with] childbirth and breastfeeding, and incised wounds. Grows in mountain valleys.

磁石

一名玄石
味辛,寒,無毒

治周痹、風濕、肢節腫痛、不可持物、洗洗酸痟,除大熱煩滿及耳聾。生山谷及山陰,有鐵處則生其陽。

---

císhí

magnetite
ALTERNATE NAME: *xuánshí* "obscure stone"
acrid flavor, cold, non-toxic

Treats all-pervasive *Bì* Impediment, wind-damp, swelling and pain in the joints of the limbs, inability to grasp things, and shivering from cold with headache;[37] and gets rid of severe heat with vexation and fullness as well as deafness. Grows in mountain valleys and on the shady side of mountains. In locations where iron is present, it grows on their sunny side.

陽起石

一名白石
味鹹,微溫,無毒

治崩中漏下,破子臟中血、癥瘕結氣,寒熱,腹痛,無子,陰痿不起,補不足。生山谷。

---

yángqǐshí

"yáng rising stone"
actinolite
ALTERNATE NAME: *báishí* "white stone"
salty flavor, slightly warm, non-toxic

Treats Center Flooding[38] and vaginal spotting; breaks up blood inside the uterus and concretions, conglomerations, and bound qì; [treats] cold and heat, abdominal pain, infertility, and Yīn Wilt with failure to raise [the penis]; and supplements insufficiency. Grows in mountain valleys.

理石

一名立制石
味辛,寒,無毒

治身熱,利胃,解煩,益精,明目,破積聚,去三蟲。生山谷。

---

lǐshí

"structurally patterned stone"
fibrous gypsum
ALTERNATE NAME: *lìzhìshí* "regulation-setting stone"
acrid flavor, cold, non-toxic

Treats generalized heat, disinhibits the stomach, resolves vexation, boosts essence, brightens the eyes, breaks up accumulations and gatherings, and gets rid of the Three Worms. Grows in mountain valleys.

長石

一名方石
味辛,寒,無毒

治身熱、四肢寒厥,利小便,通血脈,明目,去瞖眇,下三蟲,殺蠱毒。久服不飢。生山谷。

---

chángshí

"long stone"
anhydrite/feldspar
ALTERNATE NAME: *fāngshí* "square stone"
acrid flavor, cold, non-toxic

Treats generalized heat and cold reversal in the four limbs; disinhibits urination; unclogs the flow of blood in the vessels; brightens the eyes and gets rid of eye screens and one-eyed vision; moves down the Three Worms; and kills *Gǔ* Toxins. Consumed over a long time, it staves off hunger. Grows in mountain valleys.

孔公孽

一名通石
味辛,溫,無毒

治傷食不化、邪結氣、惡瘡、疽、瘻、痔,利九竅,下乳汁。生山谷。

kǒnggōngniè

"hollow old uncle sprout"
stalactite
ALTERNATE NAME: *tōngshí* "unclogging stone"[39]
acrid flavor, warm, non-toxic

Treats food damage with failure to transform [by digesting] and evil binding qì, malign sores, flat-abscesses, fistulas, and Hemorrhoids; disinhibits the Nine Orifices, and brings down the breast milk. Grows in mountain valleys.

殷孽

一名薑石
味辛,溫,無毒

治爛傷,瘀血,泄利,寒熱鼠瘻,癥瘕,結氣。生山谷及南海。

---

yīnniè

"ample sprout"
stalactite
ALTERNATE NAME: *jiāngshí* "ginger stone"
acrid flavor, warm, non-toxic

Treats putrefaction damage, static blood, diarrhea, cold and heat mouse fistulas, concretions and conglomerations, and bound blood. Grows in mountain valleys and in the far south.

中藥

Middle Medicinals

蟲部

Insects

髪髮

味苦，溫，無毒

治五癃、關格不通，利小便水道，治小兒癇、大人痓。仍自還神化。

---

fàbì

human hair
bitter flavor, warm, non-toxic

Treats the five [kinds of] *lóng* dribbling urinary stoppage and Barrier Repulsion stoppage; disinhibits urination and the waterways; treats small children's Seizures and adults' tetany. Spontaneously returns the spirit(s) and transforms.[40]

白馬莖

味鹹,平,無毒

治傷中、脈絕、陰不起,強志,益氣,長肌肉,肥健,生子。眼,平。治驚癇,腹滿,瘧疾。懸蹄,平。治驚邪、瘈瘲、乳難,辟惡氣、鬼毒、蠱疰、不祥。生平澤。

---

báimǎjīng

white horse penis
salty flavor, balanced, non-toxic

Treats damage to the center, severance of the flow in the vessels, and inability to raise the penis; strengthens the will; boosts qì; lengthens the flesh; makes you plump and healthy; and engenders offspring.[41] The eyes are balanced and treat fright Seizures, abdominal fullness, and malaria. The inside of the hooves[42] is balanced; treats fright evil, tugging and slackening, and difficulty with breastfeeding; and wards off malign qì, demon toxins, *gǔ* infixation, and bad luck. Grows in marshy flatlands.

鹿茸

味甘,溫,無毒

治漏下、惡血、寒熱、驚癇,益氣,強志,生齒,不老。角,溫,無毒。治惡瘡、癰腫,逐邪惡氣、留血在陰中。

lùróng

velvet deer antler
sweet flavor, warm, non-toxic

Treats vaginal spotting, malign blood, cold and heat, and fright Seizures; boosts qì; strengthens the will; engenders teeth; and staves off aging. The horn is warm and non-toxic. It treats malign sores and swollen welling-abscesses and drives out evil malign qì and lingering blood in the genitals.

羖羊角

味鹹,溫,無毒

治青盲,明目,殺疥蟲,止寒泄,辟惡鬼、虎、狼,止驚悖。久服安心,益氣,輕身。生川谷。

---

gǔyángjiǎo

black sheep or goat horn
salty flavor, warm, non-toxic

Treats Clear-eye Blindness; brightens the eyes; kills scabies-causing worms; stops cold diarrhea; wards off malign demons, tigers, and wolves; and stops fright palpitations. Consumed over a long time, it calms the heart, boosts qì, and lightens the body. Grows in river valleys.

牡狗陰莖

一名狗精
味鹹,平,無毒

治傷中、陰痿不起,令強熱大,生子,除女子帶下十二疾。膽,平,主明目。

mǔgǒuyīnjīng

dog penis
ALTERNATE NAME: *gǒujīng* dog essence
salty flavor, balanced, non-toxic

Treats damage to the center and Yīn Wilt with inability to raise [the penis], making it strong, hot, and large; engenders offspring; and gets rid of women's Twelve Diseases Below the Girdle. The gallbladder is balanced and indicated for brightening the eyes.

羚羊角

味鹹,寒,無毒

主明目,益氣,起陰,去惡血、注下,辟蠱毒、惡鬼、不祥,安心氣,常不魘寐。久服強筋骨,輕身。生川谷。

---

língyángjiǎo

antelope horn
salty flavor, cold, non-toxic

Indicated for brightening the eyes, boosting qì, and raising the penis; getting rid of malign blood and infixation in the lower body; warding off *Gǔ* Toxins, malign demons, and bad luck; calming heart qì; and for consistently not having nightmares. Consumed over a long period of time, it strengthens the sinews and bones and lightens the body. Grows in river valleys.

牛黃

味苦，平，有小毒

治驚癇、寒熱、熱盛、狂、痓，除邪，逐鬼。生平澤。牛角鰓，溫，無毒。下閉血，瘀血疼痛，女人帶下血。髓，補中，填骨髓，久服增年。膽，治驚，寒熱。可丸藥。

niúhuáng

"cow yellow"
cow's bezoar
bitter flavor, balanced, slightly toxic

Treats fright Seizures, cold and heat, exuberant heat, *kuáng* Mania, and tetany; expels evil; and drives out ghosts. Grows in marshy flatlands. Cow horn marrow is warm and non-toxic. It moves down blocked blood and [treats] static blood and pain, and women's vaginal discharge and bleeding. The marrow supplements the center, replenishes the marrow and brain, and increases the years when consumed over a long time. The gallbladder treats fright and cold and heat. It can be processed into a pill medication.

麝香

味辛,溫,無毒

主辟惡氣,殺鬼精物,溫瘧,蠱毒,癇,痓,去三蟲。久服除邪,不夢寤魘寐。生川谷及山中。

---

shèxiāng

"musk-deer fragrance"
musk
acrid flavor, warm, non-toxic

Indicated for warding off malign qì and killing demons and spectral entities; for warm malaria, *Gǔ* Toxins, Seizures, and tetany; and for getting rid of the Three Worms. Consumed over a long time, it gets rid of evil and staves off waking from your dreams and having nightmares. Grows in river valleys and in the mountains.

天鼠屎

一名鼠法，一名石肝
味辛，寒，無毒

治面皰腫、皮膚洗洗時痛、腹中血氣，破寒熱積聚，除驚悸。生山谷。

---

tiānshǔshǐ

bat droppings
ALTERNATE NAME: *shǔfǎ* "rat method," *shígān* "stone liver"
acrid flavor, cold, non-toxic

Treats swollen welling-abscesses in the face, shivering from cold in the skin with periodic pain, and blood and qì inside the abdomen; breaks up cold and heat accumulations and gatherings; and gets rid of fright palpitations. Grows in mountain valleys.

伏翼

一名蝙蝠
味鹹,平,無毒

治目瞑,明目,夜視有精光。久服令人喜樂,媚好,無憂。生川谷及人家室間。

---

fúyì

"crouching wings"
bat
ALTERNATE NAME: *biānfú*
salty flavor, balanced, non-toxic

Treats obscured vision, brightens the eyes, and gives night-vision and brings light into the eyeball. Consumed over a long time, it makes you joyful, charming, and worry-free. Grows in river valleys and in people's homes.

蠡魚

一名鮦魚
味甘,寒,無毒

治濕痺、面目浮腫,下大水。生池澤。

---

lí or luǒyú

northern snakehead fish
(*Ophiocephalus argus* syn. *Channa argus*)
ALTERNATE NAME: *tóngyú*
sweet flavor, cold, non-toxic

Treats damp-related *Bì* Impediment and puffy swelling in the face and around the eyes; and moves down severe water. Grows in ponds and marshes.

鯉魚膽

味苦,寒,無毒

治目熱赤痛、青盲,明目。久服強悍,益志氣。生池澤。

---

lǐyúdǎn

carp's gallbladder
bitter flavor, cold, non-toxic

Treats heat, redness, and pain in the eyes and Clear-eye Blindness; and brightens the eyes. Consumed over a long time, it makes you strong and fierce and boosts the will and qì. Grows in ponds and marshes.

烏賊魚骨

味鹹，微溫，無毒

治女子漏下赤白經汁，血閉，陰蝕腫痛，寒熱，驚氣，癥瘕，無子。生東海、池澤。

wūzéiyúgǔ

cuttlefish bone
salty flavor, slightly warm, non-toxic

Treats women's vaginal spotting in red or white and of menstrual fluid, blood block, genital erosion with swelling and pain, cold and heat, fright qì, concretions and conglomerations, and infertility. Grows in the East China Sea and in ponds and marshes.

海蛤

一名魁蛤
味苦,平,無毒

治欬逆上氣,喘息,煩滿,胸痛,寒熱。生東海。文蛤,味鹹,平,無毒。治惡瘡蝕,五痔,大孔出血。生東海,表有文。

---

hǎigé

venus clam

ALTERNATE NAME: *kuígé* "ladle clam"

bitter flavor, balanced, non-toxic

Treats counterflow cough with ascent of qì, panting, vexation and fullness, chest pain, and cold and heat. Grows in the East China Sea. The meretrix clam is salty in flavor, balanced, and non-toxic. It treats malign sores with erosion, the five [forms of] Hemorrhoids, and bleeding from large openings [in the body]. Grows in the East China Sea and has patterns on the exterior surface.

中藥 Middle Medicinals ▪ 蟲部 Insects

石龍子

一名蜥蜴
味鹹,寒,有小毒

治五癃、邪結氣,破石淋,下血,利小便水道。生川谷及山石間。

---

shílóngzǐ

"stone dragon child"
skink
ALTERNATE NAME: *xīyí* "lizard"
salty flavor, cold, slightly toxic

Treats the five [kinds of] dribbling urinary stoppage (*lóng*) and evil bound qì; breaks up stone strangury; moves down blood; and disinhibits urination and the waterways. Grows in river valleys and between rocks in the mountains.

白僵蠶

味鹹,平,無毒

治小兒驚癇、夜啼,去三蟲,滅黑䵟,令人面色好,男子陰瘍易病。生平澤。

---

báijiāngcán

infected silkworm
salty flavor, balanced, non-toxic

Treats small children's fright Seizures and crying at night, gets rid of the Three Worms, extinguishes black discoloration of the skin, causes a beautiful facial complexion, and [treats] men's yīn exchange disease. Grows in marshy flatlands.

桑螵蛸

一名蝕疣。
味鹹,平,無毒。

治傷中、疝瘕、陰痿,益精生子,女子血閉、腰痛,通五淋,利小便水道。生桑枝上。

---

sāngpíxiāo

mantis eggcase
ALTERNATE NAME: *shíyóu* "eroding warts"
salty flavor, balanced, non-toxic

Treats damage to the center, *shàn*-type ("mounding") conglomerations, and Yīn Wilt; boosts essence and engenders offspring; [treats] women's blood block and lumbar pain; unclogs the five [kinds of] strangury; and disinhibits urination and the waterways. Grows on the branches of mulberry trees.

下藥
Lower Medicinals

草部
Herbs

附子
一名茛

味辛,溫,有大毒

治風寒,咳逆,邪氣,溫中,金瘡,破癥堅、積聚、血瘕,寒濕痿躄,拘急,膝痛,不能行步。生山谷。

fùzǐ

"appended offspring"
processed offshoots of the main tuber of *Aconitum carmichaelii*[1] (monkshood/wolfsbane/aconite)
alternate name: *gèn* "Japanese buttercup"
acrid flavor, warm, highly toxic

Treats wind and cold, counterflow cough, and evil qì; warms the center; [treats] incised wounds; breaks up concretions and hardenings, gatherings and accumulations, and blood conglomerations; and [treats] cold- and damp-related crippling wilt, hypertonicity, knee pain, and inability to walk. Grows in mountain valleys.

烏頭

一名奚毒,一名即子,一名烏喙
味辛,溫,有大毒

治中風、惡風洒洒,出汗,除寒濕痺、欬逆上氣,破積聚,寒熱。其汁,煎之名射罔。殺禽獸。生山谷。

---

wūtóu

"raven-black head"
processed main tuber of *Aconitum carmichaelii*
(monkshood / wolfsbane / aconite)
ALTERNATE NAMES: *xīdú* "Tartar poison,"
jízǐ "drawing-near offspring," *wūhuì* "raven's beak"
acrid flavor, warm, highly toxic

Treats wind strike and aversion to wind with shivering from cold; brings out sweat; gets rid of cold- and damp-related *Bì* Impediment and counterflow cough with ascent of qì; breaks up accumulations and gatherings; and [treats] cold and heat. The juice, reduced by boiling, is called *shèwǎng* "shoot and ensnare." It kills wild birds and beasts. Grows in mountain valleys.

天雄

一名白幕
味辛,溫,有大毒

治大風、寒濕痹、歷節痛、拘攣緩急,破積聚,邪氣、金瘡,強筋骨,輕身,健行。生山谷。

tiānxióng

"heavenly male"
processed long tuber without offshoots of
Aconitum carmichaelii
(monkshood/wolfsbane/aconite)
ALTERNATE NAMES: : *báimù* "white curtain"
acrid flavor, warm, highly toxic

Treats great wind, cold- and damp-related *Bì* Impediment, joint-running pain, and hypertonicity and slackening and tensing; breaks up accumulations and gatherings; [treats] evil qì and incised wounds; strengthens sinews and bones; lightens the body; and makes you walk with vigor. Grows in mountain valleys.

半夏

一名地文,一名水玉
味辛,平,有毒

治傷寒寒熱、心下堅,下氣,喉咽腫痛、頭眩、胸脹、欬逆,腸鳴,止汗。生山谷。

---

bànxià

"half summer"
rhizome of *Pinellia ternata* (pinellia)
ALTERNATE NAMES: *dìwén* "earth patterns,"
shuǐyù "water jade"
acrid flavor, balanced, toxic

Treats cold damage, cold and heat, and hardness below the heart; brings down the qì; [treats] swelling and pain in the throat, dizziness in the head, distention in the chest, counterflow cough, and intestinal rumbling; and stops sweating. Grows in mountain valleys.

虎掌

味苦,溫,有大毒

治心痛、寒熱、結氣、積聚、伏梁、傷筋、痿、拘緩,利水道。生山谷。

---

hǔzhǎng

"tiger's paw"
root of *Polygonum cuspidatum* (smartweed/fleeceflower)
bitter flavor, warm, highly toxic

Treats heart pain, cold and heat, bound qì, accumulations and gatherings, Deep-Lying Beam, damage to the sinews, wilting, and [alternating] tensing and slackening; and disinhibits the waterways. Grows in mountain valleys.

鳶尾

味苦,平,有毒

治蠱毒、邪氣、鬼疰、諸毒,破癥瘕、積聚,去水,下三蟲。生山谷。

---

yuānwěi

"black kite's tail"
rhizome of *Iris tectorum* (iris)
bitter flavor, balanced, toxic

Treats *Gǔ* Toxin, evil qì, demonic infixation, and all sorts of toxins; breaks up concretions and conglomerations and accumulations and gatherings; gets rid of water; and brings down the Three Worms. Grows in mountain valleys.

大黃

味苦,寒,無毒

主下瘀血、血閉、寒熱,破癥瘕、積聚、留飲、宿食,蕩滌腸胃,推陳致新,通利水穀,調中化食,安和五臟。生山谷。

dàhuáng

"great yellow"
root of *Rheum palmatum, tanguticum*, and other species
(rhubarb)
bitter, cold, non-toxic

Indicated for bringing down static blood, blood block, and cold and heat; breaking up concretions and conglomerations, accumulations and gatherings, and lingering rheum and abiding food; scouring and flushing out the intestines and stomach; pushing out the old and making the new arrive; promoting the free passage of food and drink; attuning the center and transforming food; and calming and harmonizing the five *zàng* organs. Grows in mountain valleys.

葶藶

一名大室,一名大適
味辛,寒,無毒

治癥瘕、積聚、結氣、飲食寒熱,破堅,逐邪,通利水道。生平澤及田野。

---

tíngli

seed of *Lepidium apetalum* or *Descurainia sophia* (pepperwort)
ALTERNATE NAMES: *dàshì* "great room," *dàshì* "great fit"
acrid flavor, cold, non-toxic

Treats concretions and conglomerations, accumulations and gatherings, bound qì, and cold and heat from food and drink; breaks up firmness; drives out evil; and promotes free passage in the waterways. Grows in marshy flatlands and open fields.

草蒿

一名青蒿,一名方潰
味苦,寒,無毒

治疥瘙痂癢、惡瘡,殺蝨,留熱在骨節間,明目。生川澤。

---

cǎohāo

"field artemisia"
whole plant of *Artemisia annua* or *apiacea*
(sweet wormwood / mugwort)
ALTERNATE NAMES: *qīnghāo* "green-blue artemisia,"
fāngkuì "square bursting"
bitter flavor, cold, non-toxic

Treats itchy scabies, itchy mange, and malign sores; kills lice; [treats] lingering heat in the area of the bones and joints; and brightens the eyes. Grows in rivers and marshes.

旋覆花

一名金沸草，一名盛椹
味鹹，溫，有小毒

治結氣、脅下滿、驚悸，除水，去五臟間寒熱，補中，下氣。生平澤，川谷。

---

xuánfùhuā

"whorled upside-down flower"
flower head of *Inula britannica* or *lunariaefolia*
(yellowhead / meadow fleabane)
ALTERNATE NAMES: *jīnfèicǎo* "gold froth herb,"
shèngzhēn "exuberant mulberry fruit"
salty flavor, warm, slightly toxic

Treats bound *qì*, fullness below the rib-sides, and fright palpitations; expels water; gets rid of cold and heat in the area of the five *zàng* organs; supplements the center; and brings down the *qì*. Grows in marshy flatlands and river valleys.

藜蘆

一名蔥苒
味辛,寒,有毒

治蠱毒、欬逆、泄利、腸澼、頭瘍、疥瘙、惡瘡,殺諸蠱毒,去死肌。生山谷。

---

lílú

root and rhizome of *Veratrum nigrum* (black false hellebore)
ALTERNATE NAME: *cōngrǎn*
acrid flavor, cold, toxic

Treats *Gǔ* Toxin, counterflow cough, diarrhea, intestinal afflux, open sores on the head, itchy scabies, and malign sores; kills all sorts of *Gǔ* Toxin; and gets rid of dead flesh. Grows in mountain valleys.

鉤吻

一名野葛
味辛,溫,有大毒

治金瘡、乳痓、中惡風、欬逆上氣、水腫,殺鬼疰、蠱毒。生山谷。

---

gōuwěn

"hook kiss"
whole plant of *Gelsemium elegans* (heartbreak grass)
ALTERNATE NAME: *yěgé* "wild kudzu"
acrid flavor, warm, highly toxic

Treats incised wounds, childbed tetany, being struck by malign wind, counterflow cough with ascent of qì, and water swelling; and kills demonic infixation and *Gǔ* Toxin. Grows in mountain valleys.

射干

一名烏蒲
味苦,平,有毒

治欬逆上氣、喉痹、咽痛、不得消息,散結氣、腹中邪逆、食飲大熱。生川谷、田野。

---

shègān

"shot stem"

rhizome of *Belamcanda chinensis* (blackberry lily)

ALTERNATE NAME: *wūpú* "raven-black sweet-flag"

bitter flavor, balanced, toxic

Treats counterflow cough with ascent of qì, *Bì* Impediment in the larynx and pain in the pharynx,[2] and inability to breathe; scatters bound qì; and [treats] evil counterflow inside the abdomen and severe heat from food and drink. Grows in mountain valleys and open fields.

蛇含

一名蛇銜
味苦，微寒，無毒

治驚癇、寒熱邪氣，除熱，金瘡、疽、痔、鼠瘻、惡瘡、頭瘍。生山谷。

---

shéhán

"held in the mouth of snakes"
whole plant of *Potentilla kleiniana* (cinquefoil)
ALTERNATE NAME: *shéxián* "snake snaffle"
bitter flavor, slightly cold, non-toxic

Treats fright Seizures and the evil qì of cold and heat; expels heat; and [treats] incised wounds, flat-abscesses, Hemorrhoids, Rat Fistulas, malign sores, and open sores on the head. Grows in mountain valleys.

恆山

一名玄草
味苦,寒,有毒

治傷寒寒熱,發溫瘧,鬼毒,胸中痰結,吐逆。生川谷。

---

héngshān[3]

"perseverance mountain"
root of *Dichroa febrifuga* (dichroa root)
ALTERNATE NAME: *xuáncǎo* obscure herb
bitter flavor, cold, toxic

Treats cold damage with [alternating] cold and heat; causes warm malaria to break out; and [treats] demonic toxin, phlegm binding inside the chest, and counterflow vomiting. Grows in river valleys.

蜀漆

味辛,平,有毒

治瘧及欬逆,寒熱,腹中癥堅,痞結,積聚,邪氣,蠱毒,鬼疰。生川谷。

---

shǔqī

"lacquer from Western Sìchuān"
foliage of *Dichroa febrifuga* (dichroa leaf)
acrid flavor, balanced, toxic

Treats malaria with counterflow cough, cold and heat, concretions and firmness inside the abdomen, *pǐ* glomus binds, accumulations and gatherings, evil qì, Gǔ Toxin, and demonic infixation. Grows in river valleys.

甘遂

一名主田
味苦，寒，有毒

治大腹疝瘕、腹滿、面目浮腫、留飲、宿食，破癥堅積聚，利水穀道。生川谷。

---

gānsuì

"sweet compliance"
root of *Euphorbia kansui*
ALTERNATE NAME: *zhǔtián* "ruler of the fields"
bitter flavor, cold, toxic

Treats *shàn*-type ("mounding") conglomerations in the greater abdomen, abdominal fullness, puffy swelling in the face and eyes, lingering rheum, and abiding food; breaks up concretions and firmness and accumulations and gatherings; and disinhibits the pathways for solid and liquid food. Grows in river valleys.

白蘞

一名菟核,一名白草
味苦,平,無毒

治癰腫、疽、瘡,散結氣,止痛,除熱,目中赤,小兒驚癇,溫瘧,女子陰中腫痛。生山谷。

---

báiliǎn

"white creeper"
root of *Ampelopsis japonica* (Japanese peppervine)
ALTERNATE NAMES: *tùhé* "dodder pit," *báicǎo* "white herb"
bitter flavor, balanced, non-toxic

Treats swollen welling-abscesses and flat-abscesses, and sores; scatters bound qì; stops pain; expels heat; and [treats] redness in the center of the eyes, small children's fright Seizures, warm malaria, and women's swelling and pain inside the genitals. Grows in mountain valleys.

青葙子

一名草蒿,一名萋蒿
味苦,微寒,無毒

治邪氣、皮膚中熱、風瘙身癢,殺三蟲。
子,名草決明,治唇口青。生平谷道旁。

--- ∽ ---

qīngxiāngzǐ

seed of *Celosia argentea* (feather cockscomb)
ALTERNATE NAMES: *cǎohāo*[4] "field artemisia,"
qīhāo "luxuriant artemisia"
bitter flavor, slightly cold, non-toxic

Treats evil qì, heat inside the skin, and wind itch with generalized itching; and kills the Three Worms. The seeds are called field *juémíng* (fetid cassia) and treat green-blue lips and mouth. Grows in flatland valleys alongside roads.

蓶菌

一名蓶蘆
味鹹,平,有小毒

治心痛,溫中,去長蟲、白癬、蟯蟲、蛇螫毒、癥瘕、諸蟲。生東海池澤及勃海。

---

guànjūn[5]

"stork mushroom"
ALTERNATE NAME: *guànlú* "stork reed"
salty flavor, balanced, slightly toxic

Treats heart pain; warms the center; and gets rid of Longworms, white lichen, pinworm, snake bite poison, concretions and conglomerations, and all sorts of worms. Grows in the ponds and marshes of the East China Sea and in Bóhǎi.

白及

一名甘根，一名連及草
味苦，平，無毒

治癰腫，惡瘡，敗疽，傷陰，死肌，胃中邪氣，賊風，鬼擊，痱緩不收。生川谷。

---

báijí

"white reaching"
rhizome of *Bletilla striata* (urn orchid)
ALTERNATE NAMES: *gāngēn* "sweet root,"
liánjícǎo "connecting herb"
bitter flavor, balanced, non-toxic

Treats swollen welling-abscesses, malign sores, decaying flat-abscesses, damage to yīn, dead flesh, evil qì inside the stomach, Bandit Wind, demonic assault, and *féi* disablement with laxness and inability to contract [the four limbs]. Grows in river valleys.

大戟

一名邛鉅
味苦,寒,有小毒

治蠱毒,十二水,腹滿急痛,積聚,中風,皮膚疼痛,吐逆。

---

dàjǐ

"great halberd"
root of *Euphorbia pekinensis*[6] (Peking spurge)
ALTERNATE NAME: *qióngjù* "hillock fish-hook"
bitter flavor, cold, slightly toxic

Treats *Gǔ* Toxin; [moves down] the twelve [kinds of] water [disease]; and [treats] abdominal fullness with tension pain, accumulations and gatherings, wind strike, pain in the skin, and counterflow vomiting.

澤漆

味苦，微寒，無毒

治皮膚熱，大腹水氣，四肢面目浮腫，丈夫陰氣不足。生川澤。

---

zéqī

"marsh lacquer"
whole plant of *Euphorbia helioscopia* (sun spurge)
bitter flavor, slightly cold, non-toxic

Treats heat in the skin, water qì in the greater abdomen, puffy swelling in the four limbs and face and eyes, and insufficiency of yīn qì in men. Grows in rivers and marshes.

茵芋

味苦,溫,有毒

治五臟邪氣,心腹寒熱,羸瘦,如瘧狀發作有時,諸關節風濕痹痛。 生川谷。

---

yīnyù

foliage and stalk of *Skimmia reevesiana* (skimmia)
bitter flavor, warm, toxic

Treats evil qì in the five *zàng* organs, cold and heat in the heart and abdomen, marked emaciation, a malaria-like presentation with regularly-timed outbreaks, and wind- and damp-related *Bì* Impediment with pain in the various joints. Grows in river valleys.

貫眾

一名貫節,一名貫渠,一名百頭,
一名虎卷,一名扁符
味苦,微寒,有毒

治腹中邪熱氣、諸毒,殺三蟲。生山谷。

guànzhòng

"threaded-together multitudes"
rhizome of several different genera of fern,[7]
especially *Dryopteris crassirhizoma* (shield fern)
ALTERNATE NAMES: *guànjié* "threaded-together nodes,"
guànqú "threaded-together trench," *bǎitóu* "hundred head,"
hǔjuàn "tiger scroll," *biǎnfú* "flat Solanum"
bitter flavor, slightly cold, toxic

Treats evil heat qì inside the abdomen and all sorts of toxins, and kills the Three Worms. Grows in mountain valleys.

蕘花

味苦,寒,有毒

治傷寒、溫瘧,下十二水,破積聚大堅、癥瘕,蕩滌腸胃中留癖飲食、寒熱邪氣,利水道。生川谷。

---

yáohuā / *ráohuā*

"stubble flower"
flowers of *Wikstroemia canescens* (Himalayan tie bush)
bitter flavor, cold, toxic

Treats cold damage and warm malaria; moves down the twelve [kinds of] water [disease]; breaks up accumulations and gatherings, great firmness, and concretions and conglomerations; scours and flushes out lingering *Pǐ* Aggregations, food, and drink, and the evil qì of cold and heat; and disinhibits the waterways. Grows in river valleys.

牙子

一名狼牙
味苦,寒,有毒

治邪氣、熱氣、疥瘙、惡瘍、瘡、痔,去白蟲。生川谷。

---

yázǐ

"tooth offspring"
root of a plant tentatively identified as *Potentilla cryptotaenia*[8]
ALTERNATE NAME: *lángyá* "wolf tooth"
bitter flavor, cold, toxic

Treats evil qì, heat qì, itchy scabies, malign open sores, shallow skin disorders, and Hemorrhoids; and gets rid of Whiteworms. Grows in river valleys.

羊躑躅

味辛,溫,有大毒

治賊風皮膚中淫淫痛,溫瘧,惡毒,諸痹。生川谷。

---

yángzhízhú

"goat loitering"
flower of *Rhododendron molle* (Chinese azalea)
acrid flavor, warm, highly toxic

Treats Bandit Wind with a feeling of wantonly spreading pain inside the skin, warm malaria, malign toxins, and the various kinds of *Bì* Impediment. Grows in river valleys.

芫花

一名去水
味辛，溫，有小毒

治欬逆上氣、喉鳴、喘、咽腫、短氣、蠱毒、鬼瘧、疝瘕、癰腫，殺蟲、魚。生川谷。

---

yuánhuā

flower of *Daphne genkwa* (lilac daphne)
ALTERNATE NAME: *qùshuǐ* "get rid of water"
acrid flavor, warm, slightly toxic

Treats counterflow cough with ascent of qì, rale in the throat, panting, swollen pharynx, shortness of breath, Gǔ Toxin, demonic malaria, *shàn*-type ("mounding") conglomerations, and swollen welling-abscesses; and kills worms and fish. Grows in river valleys.

商陸

一名募根
味辛,平,有毒

治水脹、疝瘕、痹,熨除癰腫,殺鬼精物。生川谷。

---

shānglù

"Shāng mainland"
root of *Phytolacca acinosa* (India pokeweed)
ALTERNATE NAME: *tānggēn* "pokeweed root"
acrid flavor, balanced, toxic

Treats water distention, *shàn*-type ("mounding") conglomerations, and *Bì* Impediment; gets rid of swollen welling-abscesses when applied as a hot compress; and kills demons and spectral entities. Grows in river valleys.

羊蹄

一名東方宿，一名連蟲陸，一名鬼目
味苦，寒，無毒

治頭禿、疥瘙，除熱、女子陰蝕。生川澤。

---

yángtí

"goat/sheep hoof"
root of *Rumex japonicus* or *nepalensis*
(Japanese or Nepalese dock)

ALTERNATE NAMES:
dōngfāngsù "eastern direction lodge,"
liánchónglù "connecting insects mainland,"
guǐmù "ghost eye"
bitter flavor, cold, non-toxic

Treats baldness and itchy scabies and eliminates heat and women's genital erosion. Grows in rivers and marshes.

萹蓄

一名萹竹
味苦,平,無毒

治浸淫、疥瘙、疽、痔,殺三蟲。生山谷。

---

biānxù

whole plant of *Polygonum aviculare* (knotgrass/pinkweed)
ALTERNATE NAME: *biānzhú*
bitter flavor, balanced, non-toxic

Treats Wet Spreading Sores, itchy scabies, flat-abscesses, and Hemorrhoids; and kills the Three Worms. Grows in mountain valleys.

狼毒

一名續毒
味辛,平,有大毒

治欬逆上氣,破積聚,飲食寒熱,水氣,惡瘡,鼠瘻,疽蝕,鬼精,蠱毒,殺飛鳥走獸。生山谷。

---

lángdú

"wolf poison"
root of *Stellera chamaejasme*[9] (stellera)
ALTERNATE NAME: *xùdú* "reconnecting poison"
acrid flavor, balanced, highly toxic

Treats counterflow cough with ascent of qì; breaks up accumulations and gatherings; [treats] cold and heat from food and drink, water qì, malign sores, Rat Fistulas, flat-abscesses and erosion, demons and specters, and *Gǔ* Toxin, and kills flying birds and running beasts. Grows in mountain valleys.

鬼臼

一名爵犀，一名馬目毒公，一名九臼
味辛，溫，有毒

主殺蠱毒、鬼疰、精物，辟惡氣、不祥，
逐邪，解百毒。生山谷。

---

guǐjiù

"demon mortar"
root and rhizome of *Dysosma versipellis*
ALTERNATE NAMES: *juéxī* "noble rhinoceros," *mǎmùdúgōng*
"Duke Horse-Eye Poison," *jiǔjiù* "nine mortars"
acrid flavor, warm, toxic

Indicated for killing *Gǔ* Toxin, demonic infixation, spectral beings; warding off malign qì and bad luck; driving out evil; and resolving the hundred toxins. Grows in mountain valleys.

白頭翁

一名野丈人,一名胡王使者
味苦,溫,有毒

治溫瘧、狂易、寒熱、癥瘕積聚、癭氣,逐血,止痛,治金瘡。生山谷及田野。

---

báitóuwēng

"white-haired elder"
root of *Pulsatilla chinensis* (Chinese pasqueflower / anemone)
ALTERNATE NAMES: *yězhàngren* "wild father-in-law,"
húwángshǐzhě "emissary from the King
of the Northwestern tribes"
bitter flavor, warm, toxic

Treats warm malaria, rabid *kuáng* Mania, cold and heat, concretions and conglomerations and accumulations and gatherings, and goiter qì; drives out [old] blood; stops pain; and treats incised wounds. Grows in mountain valleys and open fields.

羊桃

一名鬼桃，一名羊腸
味苦，寒，有毒

治燥熱、身暴赤色、風水、積聚、惡瘍，
除小兒熱。生山林川谷及田野。

---

yángtáo[10]

"sheep/goat peach"
root of *Actinidia chinensis* (Chinese gooseberry)
ALTERNATE NAMES: *guǐtáo* "demon peach,"
yángcháng "sheep/goat intestine"
bitter flavor, cold, toxic

Treats blazing heat, generalized fulminant red color, Wind Water, accumulations and gatherings, and malign open sores; and expels heat in small children. Grows in mountain forests, river valleys, and open fields.

女青

一名雀瓢
味辛,平,有毒

治蠱毒,逐邪惡氣,殺鬼、溫瘧,辟不祥。生山谷。

---

nǚqīng[11]

"female green-blue"
ALTERNATE NAME: *quèpiáo* "sparrow calabash"
acrid flavor, balanced, toxic

Treats *Gǔ* Toxin, drives out evil malign qì, kills demons and warm malaria, and wards off bad luck. Grows in mountain valleys.

連翹

一名異翹,一名蘭華,一名折根,
一名軹,一名三廉
味苦,平,無毒

治寒熱,鼠瘻,瘰癧,癰腫,惡瘡,癭瘤,結熱,蠱毒。生山谷。

---

liánqiáo

"linked tailfeathers"
capsule of *Forsythia suspensa*
(weeping forsythia / golden bell)
ALTERNATE NAMES: *yìqiáo* "strange tailfeathers,"
lánhuā "eupatorium flower," *zhégēn* "break root,"
zhǐ "wheel-hub," *sānlián* "triple corner"
bitter flavor, balanced, non-toxic

Treats cold and heat, Rat Fistulas, scrofula, swollen welling-abscesses, malign sores, goiters and tumors of the neck, bound heat, and *Gǔ* Toxin. Grows in mountain valleys.

石下長卿

一名徐長卿
味鹹，平，有毒

治鬼疰精物、邪惡氣，殺百精，蠱毒，老魅，注易，亡走，啼哭，悲傷恍惚。生池澤、山谷。

---

shíxiàchángqīng

"under the rock leader of the stewards"
root and rhizome of *Cynanchum paniculatum* [12]
ALTERNATE NAME: *xúchāngqīng* "staid leader of the stewards"
salty flavor, balanced, toxic

Treats demonic infixation, spectral entities, and evil malign qì; kills the hundred specters; and [treats] *Gǔ* Toxin, old bogies, rabid *kuáng* Mania[13] with running around erratically and crying and wailing, and dazed absentmindedness after damaging grieving. Grows in ponds and marshes and in mountain valleys.

藺茹

味辛，寒，有小毒

主蝕惡肉、敗瘡、死肌，殺疥蟲，排膿、惡血，除大風、熱氣，善忘，不樂。生山谷。

---

lǔrú[14]

acrid flavor, cold, slightly toxic

Indicated for eroding malign flesh, putrefying wounds, and dead flesh; kills scabies-causing worms; pushes out pus and malign blood; expels great wind and heat qì; and [treats] forgetfulness and lack of joy. Grows in mountain valleys.

烏韭

味甘，寒，無毒

治皮膚往來寒熱，利小便膀胱氣。生山谷石上。

---

wūjiǔ

"raven-black allium"
whole plant or rhizome of *Stenoloma chusanum*[15] (lace fern)
sweet flavor, cold, non-toxic

Treats coming and going cold and heat in the skin and disinhibits urination and bladder qì. Grows in mountain valleys on top of rocks.

鹿藿

味苦,平,無毒

治蠱毒,女子腰腹痛,不樂,腸癰,瘰癧,瘍氣。生山谷。

---

lùhuò

"deer legume leaves"
leaves and stalk of *Rhynchosia volubilis* (snoutbean)
bitter flavor, balanced, non-toxic

Treats *Gǔ* Toxin, women's lumbar and abdominal pain, lack of joy, intestinal welling-abscesses, scrofula, and the qì of open sores. Grows in mountain valleys.

蚤休

一名蚩休
味苦,微寒,有毒

治驚癎、搖頭、弄舌、熱在腹中、癲疾、癰瘡、陰蝕,下三蟲,去蛇毒。生川谷。

---

zǎoxiū

"fleas desist"
rhizome of *Paris polyphylla* (multi-leafed paris)
ALTERNATE NAME: *chīxiū* "Chī-monster desist"
bitter flavor, slightly cold, toxic

Treats fright Seizures with shaking of the head and protruding tongue, heat inside the abdomen, Epilepsy,[16] welling-abscess sores, and genital erosion; moves the Three Worms down; and gets rid of snake toxin. Grows in river valleys.

石長生

一名丹草
味鹹，微寒，有毒

治寒熱、惡瘡、大熱，辟鬼氣、不祥。生山谷。

---

shíchángshēng

"stone life-prolonger"
whole herb of *Adiantum monochlamys*
(single-sorus maidenhair fern)
ALTERNATE NAME: *dāncǎo* "cinnabar herb"
salty flavor, slightly cold, toxic

Treats cold and heat, malign sores, and great heat; and wards off demonic qì and bad luck. Grows in mountain valleys.

藎草

味苦,平,無毒

治久欬上氣、喘逆、久寒、驚悸、痂疥、白禿、瘍氣,殺皮膚小蟲。生川谷。

jìncǎo

whole plant of *Arthraxon hispidus*
(small carpgrass a.k.a. joint-head grass)
bitter flavor, balanced, non-toxic

Treats chronic cough with ascent of qì, counterflow panting, chronic cold, fright palpitations, mange and scabies, White Balding, and the qì of open sores; and kills small worms in the skin. Grows in river valleys.

牛扁

味苦,微寒,無毒

治身皮瘡熱氣,可作浴湯,殺牛蝨、小蟲,又治牛病。生川谷。

---

niúbiǎn

"cow flat"
root, stalk, and leaves of *Aconitum ochranthum*
bitter flavor, slightly cold, non-toxic

Treats sores and heat qì in the skin all over the body, [for which purpose] it can be prepared as a medicinal bath; kills cow lice and small worms;[17] and treats bovine diseases. Grows in river valleys.

夏枯草

一名夕句、一名乃東
味苦、辛,寒,無毒

治寒熱瘰癧、鼠瘻、頭瘡,破癥,散癭結氣、腳腫、濕痹,輕身。生川谷。

---

xiàkūcǎo

"summer withering herb"
flowering part of *Prunella vulgaris*
(self-heal spike a.k.a. heal-all)
ALTERNATE NAMES: xīgōu "twilight hook,"
nǎidōng "then east"
bitter and acrid flavor, cold, non-toxic

Treats cold and heat scrofula, Rat Fistulas, and sores on the head; breaks up concretions; scatters the bound qì of goiters, swelling in the feet, and damp-related *Bì* Impediment; and lightens the body. Grows in river valleys.

敗醬

一名鹿腸
味苦，平，無毒

治暴熱，火瘡赤氣，疥瘙，疽，痔，馬鞍熱氣。生川谷。

---

bàijiàng

"rotten sauce"

whole plant with roots of *Patrinia villosa* or *P. scabiosaefolia*

ALTERNATE NAME: *lùcháng*[18] "deer intestine"

bitter flavor, balanced, non-toxic

Treats fulminant heat, the red qì of Fire Sores,[19] itchy scabies, flat-abscesses, Hemorrhoids, and the hot qì of saddles. Grows in river valleys.

白薇

味苦,平,無毒

治暴中風,身熱,肢滿,忽忽不知人,狂惑,邪氣,寒熱,酸疼,溫瘧灑灑,發作有時。生平原、川谷。

---

báiwēi

"white vetch"
root of *Cynanchum atratum* or *C. versicolor* (black swallow)
bitter flavor, balanced, non-toxic

Treats fulminant wind strike, generalized heat, fullness in the limbs, obliviousness and inability to recognize people, *kuáng* Mania and delusion, evil qì, cold and heat, soreness, and warm malaria with shivering from cold and regular outbreaks. Grows in plains and river valleys.

積雪草

味苦,寒,無毒

治大熱,惡瘡,癰疽,浸淫,赤熛,皮膚赤,身熱。生川谷。

---

jīxuěcǎo

"snow-collecting herb"
whole plant of *Centella asiatica* (gotu kola)
bitter flavor, cold, non-toxic

Treats great heat, malign sores, welling- and flat-abscesses, Wet Spreading Sores, red blaze,[20] redness in the skin, and generalized heat. Grows in river valleys.

蜀羊泉

味苦,微寒,無毒

治頭禿,惡瘡,熱氣,疥瘙,痂癬蟲,齲齒。生川谷。

---

shǔyángquán

"Western Sìchuān sheep/goat spring"
close relative of *Solanum lyratum* (lyreleaf nightshade)
bitter flavor, slightly cold, non-toxic

Treats baldness, malign sores, heat qì, itchy scabies, mange and lichen worms, and decaying teeth. Grows in river valleys.

下藥

LOWER MEDICINALS

木部

TREES

巴豆

一名巴菽
味辛,溫,有大毒

治傷寒、溫瘧、寒熱,破癥瘕、結聚堅積、留飲痰癖、大腹水脹,蕩滌五臟六腑,開通閉塞,利水穀道,去惡肉,除鬼毒、蠱疰邪物,殺蟲、魚。生川谷。

bādòu

"Eastern Sìchuān bean"
seed of *Croton tiglium* (purging croton)
ALTERNATE NAME: *bāshū* "Eastern Sìchuān legume"
acrid flavor, warm, highly toxic

Treats cold damage, warm malaria, and cold and heat; breaks up concretions, conglomerations, bindings, gatherings, firmness, and accumulations, lingering phlegm-rheum *Pǐ* Aggregations, and water distention in the greater abdomen; scours and flushes out the five *zàng* and six *fǔ* organs; unclogs blockages and congestion; disinhibits the pathways for water and grain; gets rid of malign flesh; expels demonic toxin, *gǔ* infixation, and evil entities; and kills worms and fish. Grows in river valleys.

蜀椒

味辛,溫,有毒

治邪氣、欬逆,溫中,逐骨節皮膚死肌、寒濕痺痛,下氣。久服之,頭不白,輕身,增年。生川谷。

---

shǔjiāo

"Western Sìchuān pepper"
seed capsules of *Zanthoxylum bungeanum*[21]
(Sìchuān prickly ash, a.k.a. Sìchuān peppercorn)
acrid flavor, warm, toxic

Treats evil qì and counterflow cough; warms the center; drives out [cold][22] from inside the bones, joints, and skin; gets rid of dead flesh and cold- and damp-related *Bì* Impediment with pain; and moves qì down. Consumed over a long time, it staves off whitening of the [hair on the] head, lightens the body, and increases the years. Grows in river valleys.

皂莢

味辛、鹹,溫,有小毒

治風痺、死肌、邪氣、風頭、淚出,利九竅,殺精物。生川谷。

---

zàojiá

"soap pod"
fruit of *Gleditsia sinensis* (Chinese honey locust)
acrid and salty flavor, warm, slightly toxic

Treats wind-related *Bì* Impediment, dead flesh, evil qì, wind head, and tearing; disinhibits the Nine Orifices; and kills spectral entities. Grows in river valleys.

楝實

味苦,寒,有小毒

治溫疾、傷寒、大熱、煩狂,殺三蟲、疥、瘍,利小便水道。生山谷。

---

liànshí

"Chinaberry tree fruit"[23]
fruit of *Melia toosendan* (toosendan)
bitter flavor, cold, slightly toxic

Treats acute warm conditions, cold damage, great heat, and vexation and *kuáng* Mania; kills the Three Worms, scabies, and open sores; and disinhibits urination and the waterways. Grows in mountain valleys.

鬱李仁

一名爵李
味酸，平，無毒

治大腹水腫、面目四肢浮腫，利小便水道。根，治齒齦腫、齲齒，堅齒。生高山川谷及丘陵。

---

yùlǐrén

"constrained cherry kernel"
seed of *Prunus japonica* or *P. humilis*
(oriental bush cherry or humble bush cherry)
ALTERNATE NAME: *juélǐ* "beaker cherry"
sour flavor, balanced, non-toxic

Treats water swelling in the greater abdomen and puffy swelling in the face, eyes, and four limbs; and disinhibits urination and the waterways. The roots treat swelling of the gums and decaying teeth, and hardens the teeth. Grows in high mountain river valleys and on hills.

莽草

味辛，溫，有毒

治頭風、癰腫、乳癰、疝瘕，除結氣、疥瘙，殺蟲、魚。生山谷。

---

măngcăo

"tight-clumping herb"
leaves of *Illicium lanceolatum* (Guandong star anise)
acrid flavor, warm, toxic

Treats head wind, swollen welling-abscesses, welling-abscesses in the breast, and *shàn*-type ("mounding") conglomerations; gets rid of bound qì and itchy scabies; and kills worms and fish. Grows in mountain valleys.

雷丸

一名雷矢
味苦，寒，有小毒

主殺三蟲，逐毒氣、胃中熱，利丈夫，不利女子。作膏摩，除小兒百病。生山谷土中。

léiwán

"thunder pill"
fruit of *Laccocephalum mylittae*[24]
(native bread or blackfellow's bread)
ALTERNATE NAME: *léishǐ* "thunder arrow"
bitter flavor, cold, slightly toxic

Indicated for killing the Three Worms, driving out toxic qì and heat inside the stomach. It is beneficial for men[25] but not for women. Prepared as a salve to apply by rubbing, it gets rid of the hundred diseases of small children. Grows in the soil in mountain valleys.

梓白皮

味苦,寒,無毒

治熱,去三蟲。花、葉,搗敷豬瘡。飼豬,肥大三倍。生山谷。

---

zǐbáipí

"catalpa white bark"
bark of *Catalpa ovata* (Chinese catalpa)
bitter flavor, cold, non-toxic

Treats heat and gets rid of the Three Worms. The flowers and leaves can be pounded and spread on the sores of pigs. When pigs are fed [catalpa leaves], they triple in size. Grows in mountain valleys.

桐葉

味苦,寒,無毒

治惡蝕瘡著陰。皮,治五痔,殺三蟲。花,主敷豬瘡。飼豬,肥大三倍。生山谷。

---

tóngyè

"paulownia leaf"
leaves of *Paulownia fortunei* or *P. tomentosa*
(princess tree or dragon tree)
bitter flavor, cold, non-toxic

Treats malign erosion sores attached to the genitals. The bark treats the five [types of] Hemorrhoids and kills the Three Worms. The flowers are indicated for spreading on the sores of pigs. When pigs are fed [paulownia leaves], they triple in size. Grows in mountain valleys.

藥實根

一名連木
味辛,溫,無毒

治邪氣、諸痹疼酸,續絕傷,補骨髓。生山谷。

---

yàoshígēn

"medicinal repletion root"
root of an unknown substance[26]
ALTERNATE NAME: *liánmù* "connecting wood"
acrid flavor, warm, non-toxic

Treats evil qì and all forms of *Bì* Impediment with soreness; reconnects damage from severance; and supplements bone marrow. Grows in mountain valleys.

黃環

一名凌泉，一名大就
味苦，平，有毒

治蠱毒、鬼疰、鬼魅、邪氣在臟中，除欬逆、寒熱。生山谷。

---

huánghuán

"Yellow ring"
flower of *Wisteria sinensis* [27]
ALTERNATE NAMES: *língquán* "iced-up spring,"
dàjiù "great attainment"
bitter flavor, balanced, toxic

Treats *Gǔ* Toxin, demonic infixation, ghosts and bogies, and evil qì inside the *zàng* organs; and gets rid of counterflow cough and cold and heat. Grows in mountain valleys.

溲疏

味辛,寒,無毒

治身皮膚中熱,除邪氣,止遺溺。生川谷及田野故丘墟地。可作浴湯。

---

sōushū

"urination spaced apart"
fruit of *Deutzia scabra* (fuzzy deutzia)
acrid flavor, cold, non-toxic

Treats heat in the skin all over the body, expels evil qì, and stops urinary incontinence. Grows in river valleys as well as in open fields, old burial mounds, and abandoned places. Can be prepared as a medicinal bath.

鼠李

味苦,微寒,無毒

治寒熱,療瘰瘡。生田野。

---

shǔlǐ

"rat cherry"
fruit of *Rhamnus davurica* (Dahurian buckthorn)
bitter flavor, slightly cold, non-toxic

Treats cold and heat, and scrofula and open sores. Grows in open fields.

下藥

Lower Medicinals

穀部

Food Crops

桃核仁

味苦,平,無毒

治瘀血、血閉瘕、邪氣,殺小蟲。桃花,殺疰惡鬼,令人好顏色。桃梟,在樹不落,微溫。主殺百鬼精物。桃毛,平。主下血瘕,寒熱,積聚,無子。挑蠹,殺鬼,辟邪惡、不祥。生川谷。

táohérén

seed of *Prunus persica* or *P. davidiana* (peach seed)
bitter flavor, balanced, non-toxic

Treats static blood, blood block and conglomerations, and evil qì; and kills small worms. Peach blossoms kill infixation with malign demons and gives people a beautiful complexion. Overwintered dried peaches, which have stayed on the tree without dropping, are slightly warm. They are indicated for killing the hundred demons and spectral entities. Peach fuzz is balanced. It is indicated for moving down blood conglomerations, cold and heat, and accumulations and gatherings; and for infertility. Peach moths kill demons and ward off evil, malignity, and bad luck. Grows in river valleys.

杏核仁

味甘,溫,有毒

治欬逆上氣、腸中雷鳴、喉痹,下氣,產乳,金瘡,寒心,奔豚。生川谷。

---

xìnghérén

seed of *Prunus armeniaca* (apricot seed)
sweet, warm, toxic

Treats counterflow cough with ascent of qì, rumbling sounds in the intestines, and *Bì* Impediment in the throat; moves down qì; and [is indicated for] childbirth and breastfeeding [problems], incised wounds, cold in the heart, and Bolting Piglet. Grows in river valleys.

假蘇

一名鼠蓂
味辛，溫，無毒

治寒熱、鼠瘻、瘰癧生瘡，破結聚氣，下瘀血，除濕痹。生川澤。

---

jiǎsū

"false perilla"
whole herb of *Schizonepeta tenuifolia*[28] (Japanese catnip)
ALTERNATE NAME: *shǔmò* "rat solitude"
acrid flavor, warm, non-toxic

Treats cold and heat, Rat Fistulas, and scrofula with the formation of sores; breaks up binding and gathering qì; moves down static blood; and expels damp-related *Bì* Impediment. Grows in rivers and marshes.

苦瓠

味苦，寒，有毒

治大水、面目四肢浮腫，下水，令人吐。
生川澤。

---

kǔhù

"bitter calabash"
fruit of *Lagenaria siceraria var. gourda* (bottlegourd)
bitter flavor, cold, toxic

Treats great water and puffy swelling in the face, eyes, and four limbs; moves down water; and makes people vomit. Grows in rivers and marshes.

大豆黃卷

味甘,平,無毒

治濕痹,筋攣,膝痛。生大豆,平。塗癰腫。煮汁飲,殺鬼毒,止痛。赤小豆,平。主下水,排癰腫膿血。生平澤。

---

dàdòuhuángjuǎn

"soybean yellow curls"
sprouted seed of *Glycine max*[29] (dried soybean sprouts)
sweet flavor, balanced, non-toxic

Treats damp-related *Bì* Impediment, hypertonicity of the sinews, and knee pain. Raw soybeans are balanced. Rub them on swollen welling-abscesses. Decocting them and drinking the liquid kills demon toxin and stops pain. "Small red beans"[30] are balanced. They are indicated for moving water down and pushing out the pus and blood of swollen welling-abscesses. Grows in marshy flatlands.

腐婢

小豆花也
味辛,平,無毒

治痎瘧,寒熱,邪氣,泄利,陰不起,病酒頭痛。

---

fǔbì

"rotten slave girl"
(bean flowers)[31]
This means the flowers of small beans.
acrid flavor, balanced, non-toxic

Treats malaria, cold and heat, evil qì, diarrhea, inability to raise the penis, and alcohol-induced headaches.

下藥

Lower Medicinals

石部

Rocks

石膽

一名畢石
味酸,寒,有毒

主明目,目痛,金瘡,諸癎,痙,女子陰蝕痛,石淋,寒熱,崩中下血,諸邪毒氣,令人有子。煉餌服之,不老。久服,增壽,神仙。能化鐵為銅,成金銀。生山谷大石間。

---

shídǎn

"stone gall"
chalcanthite (blue vitriol)
ALTERNATE NAME: *bìshí* "net stone"
sour flavor, cold, toxic

Indicated for brightening the eyes, eye pain, incised wounds, all types of Seizures, tetany, women's genital erosion and pain, stone stranguary, cold and heat, Center Flooding and [vaginal] bleeding, all kinds of evil and toxic qì, and for making people fertile. Alchemically refining this substance and ingesting it staves off aging. Consumed over a long time, it increases longevity and [turns you into] a spirit immortal. It can transform iron to make copper, and it can produce gold and silver. Grows in mountain valleys between large rocks.

雄黃

一名黃食石
味苦，平，有毒

治寒熱、鼠瘻、惡瘡、疽、痔、死肌，殺精物、惡鬼、邪氣、百蟲毒腫，勝五兵。煉食之，輕身，神仙。生山谷，山之陽。

xiónghuáng

"rooster yellow"
realgar
ALTERNATE NAME: *huángshíshí* "yellow feed stone"
bitter flavor, balanced, toxic

Treats cold and heat, Rat Fistulas, malign sores, flat-abscesses, Hemorrhoids, and dead flesh; kills spectral entities and malign demons, evil qì, and toxins from the hundred worms with swelling; and prevails over the Five Weapons.[32] Alchemically refining it and eating it lightens the body and [turns you into] a spirit immortal. Grows in mountain valleys on the south-facing side of the mountain.

雌黃

味辛,平,有毒

治惡瘡、頭禿、痂疥,殺毒蟲、蝨,身癢、邪氣、諸毒。煉之,久服輕身,增年,不老。生山谷。

---

cíhuáng

"hen yellow"
orpiment
acrid flavor, balanced, toxic

Treats malign wounds, baldness, and mange and scabies; kills poisonous worms and lice; and [treats] generalized itching, evil qì, and all kinds of toxins. Alchemically refining it and consuming it over a long time lightens the body, increases the years, and staves off aging. Grows in mountain valleys.

水銀

味辛,寒,有毒

治疥瘙、痂瘍、白禿,殺皮膚中蟲、蝨,墮胎,除熱,殺金、銀、銅、錫毒。鎔化還復為丹。久服神仙,不死。生平土,出於丹砂。

shuǐyín

"liquid silver"
mercury
acrid flavor, cold, toxic

Treats itchy scabies, mange, and White Balding; kills worms in the skin and lice; makes the fetus drop;[33] eliminates heat; kills the toxins of gold, silver, copper, and tin. Melted down it returns to its previous state of cinnabar. Consumer over a long time, it [turns you into] a spirit immortal and staves off death. Grows in flat ground and comes out of cinnabar.

膚青

一名推青
味辛,平,無毒

治蠱毒及蛇、菜、肉諸毒,惡瘡。生川谷。

---

fūqīng[34]

"skin green-blue"
ALTERNATE NAME: *tuīqīng* "push green-blue"
acrid flavor, balanced, non-toxic

Treats *Gǔ* Toxin, all kinds of poisoning from snakes, plants, and meats, and malign wounds. Grows in river valleys.

凝水石

一名白水石
味辛,寒,無毒

治身熱,腹中積聚,邪氣,皮中如火燒,煩滿。水飲之。久服不飢。生山谷。

---

níngshuǐshí

"congealed liquid stone"
glauberite
ALTERNATE NAME: *báishuǐshí* "white liquid stone"
acrid flavor, cold, non-toxic

Treats generalized heat, accumulations and gatherings in the abdomen, evil qì, a sensation like burning fire inside the skin, and vexation and fullness. Drink it down with water. Consumed over a long time, it staves off hunger. Grows in mountain valleys.

鐵落

味辛,平,無毒

治風熱,惡瘡,瘍疽瘡,痂疥氣在皮膚中。鐵精,平,主明目,化銅。鐵,主堅肌,耐痛。生平澤。

---

tiěluò

"iron drop"
iron shavings
acrid flavor, balanced, non-toxic

Treats wind heat, malign sores, open sores and flat-abscesses, and the qì of mange and scabies inside the skin. Blast furnace ash is balanced and is indicated for brightening the eyes and transforming copper. Iron is indicated for making the flesh firm and allowing you to withstand pain. Grows in marshy flatlands.

鉛丹

味辛,微寒

治吐逆、胃反、驚癇、癲疾,除熱,下氣。煉化還成九光。久服通神明。生平澤。

---

qiāndān

"lead cinnabar-red"
minium
acrid flavor, slightly cold

Treats vomiting counterflow and stomach reflux, fright Seizures, and Epilepsy; eliminates heat; and moves down the qì. When melted, it changes and returns [to its former state] and forms the Nine Radiances.[35] Consumed over a long time, it facilitates the breakthrough of spirit illumination. Grows in marshy flatlands.

粉錫

一名解錫
味辛,寒,無毒

治伏屍、毒螫,殺三蟲。錫鏡鼻,平。治女子血閉,癥瘕,伏腸,絕孕。生山谷。

---

fěnxī

"powdered tin"
white lead
ALTERNATE NAME: *jiěxī* "dismembered tin"
acrid flavor, cold, non-toxic

Treats Lurking Corpse and toxic insect stings or bites; and kills the Three Worms. Tin mirror knobs are balanced. They treat women's blood block, concretions and conglomerations, "lurking intestine,"[36] and interrupted pregnancy.[37] Grows in mountain valleys.

代赭

一名須丸
味苦,寒,無毒

治鬼疰、賊風、蠱毒,殺精物、惡鬼,腹中毒,邪氣,女子赤沃漏下。生山谷。

---

dàizhě

"substitute russet"
hematite
ALTERNATE NAME: *xūwán* "must-have pill"
bitter flavor, cold, non-toxic

Treats demonic infixation, Bandit Wind, and *Gǔ* Toxin; kills spectral entities and malign demons; [and treats] toxin inside the abdomen, evil qì, and women's red soaking and vaginal spotting. Grows in mountain valleys.

鹵鹹

一名寒石
味苦，寒，無毒

治大熱、消渴、狂煩，除邪及吐下蠱毒，柔肌膚。生鹽池。大鹽，一名胡鹽。寒，無毒。治腸胃結熱，令人吐。生池澤。戎鹽，主明目，目痛，益氣，堅肌骨，去毒蠱。生北地。

lǔxián[38]

"alkaline saltiness"
bittern deposit
ALTERNATE NAME: *hánshí* "cold stone"
bitter flavor, cold, non-toxic

Treats great heat, dispersion thirst, and *kuáng* Mania with vexation; eliminates evil and [gets rid of] *Gǔ* Toxin by elimination through vomiting or downward movement; and softens the skin and flesh. Grows in salt ponds. "Great salt" (*dàyán*) is also called "northwestern tribes salt." It is cold and non-toxic. It treats bound heat in the intestines and stomach and induces vomiting. Grows in ponds and marshes. "Western tribes salt" (*róngyán*) is indicated for brightening the eyes, for eye pain, and for boosting qì; firms the flesh and bones; and gets rid of toxic *gǔ*. Grows in the northern lands.

青琅玕

一名石珠
味辛，平，無毒

治身癢，火瘡，癰傷，白禿，疥瘙，死肌。生平澤。

---

qīnglánggān[39]

"green-blue *lánggān*"
malachite
ALTERNATE NAME: *shízhū* "stone pearl"
acrid flavor, balanced, non-toxic

Treats generalized itching, Fire Sores, damage from welling-abscesses, White Balding, itchy scabies, and dead flesh. Grows in marshy flatlands.

礜石

一名青分石,一名立制石,一名固羊石
味辛,大熱,有毒

治寒熱、鼠瘻、蝕瘡、死肌、風痹、腹中堅癖、邪氣,除熱。生山谷。

---

yùshí

"arsenic stone"
arsenopyrite
ALTERNATE NAMES: *qīngfēnshí* "greenblue division stone,"
lìzhìshí "establish and conform stone,"
gùyángshí "secure goat/sheep stone"
acrid flavor, very hot, toxic

Treats cold and heat, Rat Fistulas, erosion sores, dead flesh, wind-related *Bì* Impediment, firm *Pǐ* Aggregations in the abdomen, and evil qì, and eliminates heat. Grows in mountain valleys.

石灰

一名惡灰
味辛,溫

治疽、瘍、疥瘙、熱氣、惡瘡、癩疾、死肌墮眉,殺痔蟲,去黑子、息肉。生川谷。

---

shíhuī

"stone ash"
limestone
ALTERNATE NAME: *èhuī* "malign ash"
acrid flavor, warm[40]

Treats flat-abscesses, open sores, itchy scabies, heat qì, malign sores, and *lài* leprosy with dead flesh and loss of eyebrows; kills hemorrhoid[-causing] worms;[41] and gets rid of moles and polyps. Grows in river valleys.

白堊

味苦,溫,無毒

治女子寒熱,癥瘕,月閉,積聚,陰腫痛,漏下,無子。生山谷。

---

báiè

"white plaster"
chalk
bitter flavor, warm, non-toxic

Treats women's cold and heat, concretions and conglomerations, menstrual block, accumulations and gatherings, swelling and pain in the genitals, vaginal spotting, and infertility. Grows in mountain valleys.

冬灰

一名藜灰
味辛,微溫

治黑子,去疣、息肉、疽蝕、疥瘙。生川澤。

---

dōnghuī

"Winter ash"[42]
ALTERNATE NAME: *líhuī* "chenopodium ash"
acrid flavor, slightly warm

Treats moles; and gets rid of warts, polyps, flat-abscesses with erosion, and itchy scabies. Grows in rivers and marshes.

下藥

Lower Medicinals

蟲部

Insects

六畜毛蹄甲

味鹹，平，有毒

治鬼疰，蠱毒，寒熱，驚癇，癲，痙，狂走。駱駝毛，尤良。犀角，味苦，寒，無毒。治百毒、蠱疰、邪鬼、瘴氣，殺鉤吻、鴆羽、蛇毒，除邪，不迷惑，魘寐。久服輕身。生山谷。

---

liùchùmáotíjiǎ

hair, hooves, and nails from the six domestic animals [43]
salty flavor, balanced, toxic

Treats demonic infixation, *Gǔ* Toxin, cold and heat, fright Seizures, Epilepsy, tetany, and *kuáng* Mania with running around. Camel's hair is particularly excellent. Rhinoceros horn [44] is bitter in flavor, cold, and non-toxic. It treats the hundred toxins, *gǔ* infixation, evil demons, and Southern miasmic qì; [45] kills [poisoning from] Gōuwěn, [46] from the feathers of the zhēn bird, [47] and from snake [bites]; eliminates evil; and staves off confusion and nightmares. Consumed over a long time, it lightens the body. Grows in mountain valleys.

豚卵

一名豚顛
味甘,溫,無毒

治驚癇、癲疾、鬼疰、蠱毒,除寒熱、奔豚、五癃、邪氣、攣縮。懸蹄,平。主五痔,伏熱在腸,腸癰內蝕。

---

túnluǎn

piglet testicles
ALTERNATE NAME: *túndiān* "piglet vertex"
sweet flavor, warm, non-toxic

Treats fright Seizures, Epilepsy, demonic infixation, and *Gǔ* Toxin; eliminates cold and heat, Bolting Piglet, the five types of dribbling urinary block, evil qì, and contractures. The dewclaw is balanced. It is indicated for the five types of Hemorrhoids, for lurking heat in the intestines, and for intestinal welling-abscesses with internal erosion.

麋脂

一名官脂
味辛,溫,無毒

治癰腫,惡瘡,死肌,風寒濕痹,四肢拘緩不收,風頭腫。氣通膜理。生山谷及淮海邊。

---

mízhī

elaphure fat
ALTERNATE NAME: *guānzhī* "official's fat"
acrid flavor, warm, non-toxic

Treats swollen welling-abscesses, malign sores, dead flesh, wind-, cold-, and damp-related *Bì* Impediment, hypertonicity and slackening with paresis, and wind head with swelling. Unclogs the qì in the interstices. Grows in mountain valleys and in the Southern border regions between the Huái River and the ocean.

鼺鼠

微溫

主墮胎,令產易。生平谷。

---

léishǔ

Pteromys momonga (Japanese dwarf flying squirrel)
slightly warm

Indicated for making the fetus drop and for making childbirth easy. Grows in flatland valleys.

燕屎

味辛,平,有毒

治蠱毒、鬼疰,逐不祥、邪氣,破五癃,利小便。生高山、平谷。

---

yànshǐ

swallow droppings
acrid flavor, balanced, toxic

Treats *Gǔ* Toxin and demonic infixation; drives out bad luck and evil qì; breaks up the five [types of] dribbling urinary block; and disinhibits urination. Grows in high mountains and flatland valleys.

龜甲

一名神屋
味鹹,平,有毒

治漏下赤白,破癥瘕,痎瘧、五痔、陰蝕、濕痹、四肢重弱、小兒囟不合。久服輕身,不飢。生南海、池澤及湖水中。

---

guījiǎ

Mauremys reevesii, syn. *Chinemys reevesii*
(Reeve's turtle shell)
ALTERNATE NAME: *shénwū* "spirit residence"
salty flavor, balanced, toxic

Treats red and white vaginal spotting; breaks up concretions and conglomerations; and [treats] malaria, the five [types of] Hemorrhoids, erosion in the genitals, heaviness and weakness of the four limbs, and failure of the skull bones in small children to close. Consumed over a long time, it lightens the body and staves off hunger. Grows in ponds and marshes and in lake water in the far south.[48]

蝦蟆

味辛，寒，有毒

治邪氣，破癥堅血，癰腫，陰瘡。服之不患熱病。生江湖池澤。

---

hámá

Fejervarya limnocharis or similar species (frog or toad)
acrid flavor, cold, toxic

Treats evil qì; breaks up concretions and firmed up blood; and [treats] swollen welling-abscesses and genital sores. When you consume this substance, you will no longer be troubled by heat disorders. Grows in rivers, lakes, ponds, and marshes.

鮀魚甲

味辛，微溫，有毒

治心腹癥瘕，伏堅積聚，寒熱，女子崩中下血五色，小腹陰中相引痛，瘡疥，死肌。生南海、池澤。

---

tuóyújiǎ[49]

shell of an unknown aquatic animal
acrid flavor, slightly warm, toxic

Treats concretions and conglomerations in the heart and abdomen, lurking firmness and gathering and accumulations, cold and heat, women's Center Flooding and vaginal bleeding [and discharge] in the five colors, pain stretching from the lesser abdomen to the inside of the genitals, sores and scabies, and dead flesh. Grows in ponds and marshes in the far south.

鱉甲

味鹹,平,無毒

治心腹癥瘕堅積、寒熱,去痞、息肉、陰蝕、痔、惡肉。生池澤。

---

biējiǎ

Pelodiscus sinensis, syn. *Amyda sinensis* (softshell turtle shell)
salty flavor, balanced, non-toxic

Treats concretions, conglomerations, firmness, and accumulations in the heart and abdomen along with cold and heat; and gets rid of *pǐ* glomus, polyps, genital erosion, Hemorrhoids, and malign flesh. Grows in ponds and marshes.

蚱蟬

味鹹，寒，無毒

治小兒驚癇，夜啼，癲病，寒熱。生楊樹上。

---

zhàchán

Cryptotympana atrata and related species (black cicada)
salty flavor, cold, non-toxic

Treats small children's fright Seizures, crying at night, Epilepsy, and cold and heat. Grows on poplars.

露蜂房

一名蜂腸
味苦,平,有毒

治驚癇,瘲瘲,寒熱,邪氣,癲疾,鬼精,蠱毒,腸痔。生山谷。

---

lúfēngfáng

Polistes mandarinus[50] (paper wasp nest)
ALTERNATE NAME: *fēngcháng* "wasp intestines"
bitter flavor, balanced, toxic

Treats fright Seizures, tugging and slackening, cold and heat, evil qì, Epilepsy, demons and specters, *Gǔ* Toxin, and intestinal Hemorrhoids. Grows in mountain valleys.

馬刀

味辛,微寒,有毒

治漏下赤白、寒熱,破石淋,殺禽獸、賊鼠。生江湖池澤及東海。

---

mǎdāo

"horse knife"
Solen gouldii (razor-shell clam)
acrid flavor, slightly cold, toxic

Treats vaginal spotting in red and white, with cold and heat; breaks up stone strangury; and kills wild birds and beasts and bandit rodents. Grows in rivers, lakes, ponds, and marshes, and in the East China Sea.

蟹

味鹹，寒，有毒

治胸中邪氣，熱結痛，喎僻，面腫，敗漆。燒之致鼠。生池澤諸水中。

---

xiè

Eriocheir sinensis (Chinese mitten crab)
salty flavor, cold, toxic

Treats evil qì inside the chest, heat binding pain, deformation and distortion of the face, and swelling in the face; and defeats lacquer.[51] Burning it causes rodents to arrive.[52] Grows in ponds and marshes and all kinds of water.

蛇蛻

一名龍子衣,一名蛇符,
一名龍子單衣,一名弓皮
味鹹,平,無毒

治小兒百二十種驚癇,瘈瘲,癲疾,寒熱,腸痔,蟲毒,蛇癇。生川谷及田野。

shétuì

sloughed snake skin[53]
ALTERNATE NAMES: *lóngzǐyī* "dragon child clothes,"
shéfú "snake talisman," *lóngzǐdānyī* "dragon child garment,"
gōngpí "bow skin"
salty flavor, balanced, non-toxic

Treats the 120 kinds of fright Seizures in small children, tugging and slackening, and Epilepsy; cold and heat; intestinal Hemorrhoids; insect toxins; and Snake Seizures. Grows in river valleys and open fields.

猬皮

味苦,平,無毒

治五痔,陰蝕,下血赤白五色血汁不止,陰腫痛引腰背。酒煮殺之。生川谷、田野。

---

wèipí

hedgehog skin
bitter flavor, balanced, non-toxic

Treats the five [types of] Hemorrhoids; genital erosion; vaginal discharge of blood or of red and white fluid, or in the five colors, with incessant loss of blood; and swelling and pain in the genitals that stretches to the lumbus and back. Decocting it in liquor kills it.[54] Grows in river valleys and open fields.

蠮螉

味辛,平,無毒

治久聾,欬逆,毒氣,出刺,出汗。生川谷或人屋間。

---

yēwēng

Ammophila vagabunda or *Eumenes pomiformis* (potter wasp)
acrid flavor, balanced, non-toxic

Treats chronic deafness, counterflow cough, and toxin qì; makes thorns come out; and promotes sweating. Grows in river valleys or inside people's houses.

蜣蠅

一名蛣蜣
味鹹,寒,有毒

治小兒驚癇,瘈瘲,腹脹,寒熱,大人癲疾,狂易。生池澤。

---

qiānglánɡ

Catharsius molossus (dung beetle)
ALTERNATE NAME: : *jiéqiāng*
salty flavor, cold, toxic

Treats fright Seizures in small children, tugging and slackening, abdominal distention, and cold and heat; and Epilepsy and rabid *kuáng* Mania[55] in adults. Grows in ponds and marshes.

蛞蝓

一名陵蠡
味鹹，寒，無毒

治賊風喎僻，胅筋，及脫肛，驚癇，攣縮。生池澤及陰地、沙石、垣下。

---

kuòyú

Limax (slug)
ALTERNATE NAME: *língluó* "mound snail"
salty flavor, cold, non-toxic

Treats Bandit Wind with distorted face and protruding sinews, as well as rectal prolapse, fright Seizures, and contractures. Grows in ponds and marshes, as well as in shady soil, sand and stones, and under walls.

白頸蚯蚓

味鹹,寒,無毒

治蛇瘕,去三蟲、伏屍、鬼疰、蠱毒,殺長蟲。仍自化作水。生平土。

báijǐngqiūyǐn

Pheretima aspergillum, Allolobophora caliginosa trapezoides,
and many other species (earthworm)
salty flavor, cold, non-toxic

Treats Snake Conglomerations; gets rid of the Three Worms, Lurking Corpse, demonic infixation, and *Gǔ* Toxin; and kills Longworms. It can repeatedly transform itself into water. Grows in plains.

蠐螬

一名蟦蠐
味鹹,微溫,有毒

治惡血,血瘀,痺氣,破折,血在脅下堅滿痛,月閉,目中淫膚、青翳、白膜。生平澤及人家積糞草中。

---

qícáo

Holotrichia diomphalia (Korean black chafer)
ALTERNATE NAME: *féiqí*
salty flavor, slightly warm, toxic

Treats malign blood; blood stasis; *Bì* Impediment qì; breaks and fractures; blood below the rib-sides with firmness, fullness, and pain; menstrual block; and extra skin, green-blue screens, and white membranes in the eyes. Grows in marshy flatland and in the grasses [that grow on] accumulated human manure by people's homes.

石蠶

一名沙蝨
味鹹,寒,有毒

治五癃,破石淋,墮胎。肉,解結氣,利水道,除熱。生池澤。

---

shícán

"stone silkworm"
Phryganea japonica (Japanese caddisfly)
ALTERNATE NAME: *shāshī* "sand flea"
salty flavor, cold, toxic

Treats the five types of dribbling urinary block, breaks up stone strangury, and makes the fetus drop. The flesh resolves bound qì, disinhibits the waterways, and eliminates heat. Grows in ponds and marshes.

雀甕

一名躁舍
味甘,平,無毒

治小兒驚癇,寒熱,結氣,蠱毒,鬼疰。
生樹枝間。

---

quèwèng

"sparrow jar"
Monema flavescens a.k.a. *Cnidocampa flavescens*
(pupa of the nettle moth)
ALTERNATE NAME: *zàoshè* "sparrow's nest"
sweet flavor, balanced, non-toxic

Treats fright Seizures in small children, cold and heat, bound qì, *Gǔ* Toxin, and demonic infixation. Grows between tree branches.

樗雞

味苦,平,有小毒

治心腹邪氣、陰痿,益精,強志,生子,好色,補中,輕身。生川谷樗樹上。

---

chūjī

"ailanthus chicken"
Huechys sanguinea (black and scarlet cicada)
bitter flavor, balanced, slightly toxic

Treats evil qì in the heart and abdomen and Yīn Wilt, boosts essence, strengthens the will, engenders offspring, beautifies the complexion,[56] supplements the center, and lightens the body. Grows in river valleys on top of ailanthus trees.

斑螯

一名龍尾
味辛，寒，有毒

治寒熱、鬼疰、蠱毒、鼠瘻、惡瘡、疽、蝕、死肌，破石癃。生川谷。

---

bānmáo

Mylabris phalerata or *cichorii* (Chinese blister beetle)
ALTERNATE NAME: *lóngwěi* "dragon tail"
acrid flavor, cold, toxic

Treats cold and heat, demonic infixation, *Gǔ* Toxin, Rat Fistulas, malign sores, flat-abscesses and erosion, and dead flesh; and breaks up stone strangury. Grows in river valleys.

螻蛄

一名蟪蛄,一名天螻,一名螜
味鹹,寒,無毒

治產難,出肉中刺,潰癰腫,下哽噎,解毒,除惡瘡。生平澤。

---

lóugū

Gryllotalpa (mole-cricket)
ALTERNATE NAMES: *huìgū, tiānlóu, hú*
salty flavor, cold, non-toxic

Treats childbirth complications, makes thorns in the flesh come out, bursts swollen welling-abscesses, moves down choking obstructions in the throat, resolves toxins, and gets rid of malign sores. Grows in marshy flatlands.

蜈蚣

味辛,溫,有毒

治鬼疰、蠱毒,噉諸蛇、蟲、魚毒,殺鬼物老精、溫瘧,去三蟲。生川谷。

---

wúgōng

Scolopendra subspinipes (giant centipede,
a.k.a. Vietnamese or jungle centipede)
acrid flavor, warm, toxic

Treats demonic infixation and *Gǔ* Toxin; feeds on snake, bug, and fish toxin; kills demonic entities and old specters; [treats] warm malaria; and gets rid of the Three Worms. Grows in river valleys.

馬陸

一名百足
味辛,溫,有毒

治腹中大堅癥,破積聚,息肉,惡瘡,白禿。生川谷。

---

mǎlù

Prospirobolus joannsi (millipede)
ALTERNATE NAME: *bǎizú* "hundred feet"
acrid flavor, warm, toxic

Treats serious firmness and concretions inside the abdomen, breaks up accumulations and gatherings, and [treats] polyps, malign sores, and White Balding. Grows in river valleys.

地膽

一名蚖青
味辛,寒,有毒

治鬼疰、寒熱、鼠瘻、惡瘡、死肌,破癥瘕,墮胎。生川谷。

---

dìdǎn

"earth gall"
Meloe coarctatus (oil beetle)
ALTERNATE NAME: *yuánqīng* "newt azure"
acrid flavor, cold, toxic

Treats demonic infixation, cold and heat, Rat Fistulas, malign sores, and dead flesh; breaks up concretions and conglomerations; and makes the fetus drop. Grows in river valleys.

螢火

一名夜光
味辛,微溫,無毒

主明目,小兒火瘡,傷熱氣,蠱毒,鬼疰,通神精。生階地、池澤。

---

yínghuǒ

"glow-worm fire"
Luciola (Japanese firefly)
ALTERNATE NAME: *yèguāng* "night glow"
acrid flavor, slightly warm, non-toxic

Indicated for brightening the eyes and for small children's Fire Sores and damage from heat qì, for *Gǔ* Toxin and demonic infixation, and for facilitating the breakthrough of spirit essence.[57] Grows in terraced land and in ponds and marshes.

衣魚

一名白魚
味鹹,溫,無毒

治婦人疝瘕,小便不利,小兒中風,項強,皆宜摩之。生平澤。

---

yīyú

"clothes fish"
Lepisma saccharina (silverfish)
ALTERNATE NAME: *báiyú* "white fish"
salty flavor, warm, non-toxic

Treats women's *shàn*-type ("mounding") conglomerations and inhibited urination, and small children's wind strike and rigidity in the neck. In all cases, rub it on.[58] Grows in marshy flatlands.

鼠婦

一名負燔,一名蚜蠘
味酸,溫,無毒

治氣癃不得小便、婦人月閉、血瘕、癇、痓、寒熱,利水道。生平谷及人家地上。

---

shǔfù

Armadillidium vulgare (pill bug, a.k.a. wood louse)
ALTERNATE NAMES: *fùfán, yīqī*
sour flavor, warm, non-toxic

Treats qì dribbling urinary block and inability to urinate, women's menstrual block, blood conglomerations, Seizures, tetany, and cold and heat; and disinhibits the waterways. Grows in flat valleys and on the floor in people's homes.

水蛭

一名至掌
味鹹，平，有毒

主逐惡血、瘀血、月閉，破血瘕、積聚，無子，利水道。生池澤。

---

shuǐzhì

Hirudo nipponica and related species (leech)
ALTERNATE NAME: *zhìzhǎng* "reach the palm of the hand"
salty flavor, balanced, toxic

Indicated for driving out malign blood, static blood, and menstrual block; breaking up blood conglomerations and accumulations and gatherings; [treating] infertility; and for disinhibiting the waterways. Grows in ponds and marshes.

木蛇

一名魂常
味苦,平,有毒

治目赤痛,眥傷,淚出,瘀血,血閉,寒熱,酸瘻,無子。生川澤。

---

mùméng

"tree gadfly"
Solva tigrina or *walker* and related species (wood soldier-fly)
ALTERNATE NAME: *húncháng* "*hún* soul constant"
bitter flavor, balanced, toxic

Treats redness and pain in the eyes, damage to the corners of the eyes, tearing, static blood, blood block, cold and heat, sore and weak flesh,[59] and infertility. Grows in rivers and marshes.

蜚蟲

味苦,微溫,有毒

主逐瘀血,破下血積、堅痞癥瘕,寒熱,通利血脈及九竅。生川谷。

---

fěiméng[60]

Tabanus bivittatus (horse fly)
bitter flavor, slightly warm, toxic

Indicated for driving out static blood; breaking up and moving down blood accumulations, firmness, *pǐ* glomus, and concretions and conglomerations; [treating] cold and heat; and promoting free flow in the blood vessels and Nine Orifices. Grows in river valleys.

蜚蠊

味鹹,寒,有毒

治血瘀癥堅,寒熱,破積聚,喉咽痹,內寒無子。生川澤及人家屋間。

---

fěilián

Blatta orientalis (cockroach)
salty flavor, cold, toxic

Treats blood stasis, concretions and firmness, and cold and heat; breaks up accumulations and gatherings and *Bì* Impediment in the throat; and [treats] infertility that is [due to] internal cold. Grows in rivers and marshes and inside people's homes.

䗪蟲

一名地鱉
味鹹,寒,有毒

治心腹寒熱洗洗、血積、癥瘕,破堅,下血閉。生子大良。生川澤及沙中、人家牆壁下土中濕處。

---

zhèchóng

Eupolyphaga sinensis or *Opisthoplatia orientalis*
(wingless cockroach)
ALTERNATE NAME: *dìbiē* "earth soft-shell turtle"
salty flavor, cold, toxic

Treats cold and heat in the heart and abdomen with shivering, blood accumulations, and concretions and conglomerations; breaks up firmness; and moves down blood block. Most excellent for engendering offspring. Grows in rivers and marshes, as well as in sand and in damp places in the ground under walls in people's homes.

貝子

一名貝齒
味鹹，平，有毒

治目翳、鬼疰、腹痛，下血、五癃，利水道。生東海、池澤。

---

bèizǐ

cowrie shell
ALTERNATE NAME: *bèichǐ*
salty flavor, balanced, toxic

Treats eye screens, demonic infixation, and abdominal pain; moves down blood and the five kinds of dribbling urinary block; and disinhibits the waterways. Grows in the East China Sea and ponds and marshes.

彼子

味甘,溫,有毒

治腹中邪氣,去三蟲、蛇螫、蠱毒、鬼疰、伏屍。生山谷。

---

bǐzǐ[61]

torreya seed
sweet flavor, warm, toxic

Treats evil qì inside the abdomen; gets rid of the Three Worms and snake bite and *Gǔ* Toxin; and [treats] demonic infixation and Lurking Corpse. Grows in mountain valleys.

上藥

UPPER MEDICINALS

NOTES

1. Locally also *L. japonicus, sibiricus,* or *artemisia*.

2. *Polygala sibirica* is often used as a substitute.

3. I leave it to the reader's choice and imagination whether this expression, which I have translated literally, refers specifically to the effect of lengthening the penis or should be read in more general terms.

4. The term 精光 *jīngguāng* is often explained as referring to gleaming pupils. As an unfortunate result of the inherent vagueness of literary Chinese, it is not clear whether this gleam in the pupils was interpreted as a reflection of the state of essence in the person. In other early literature (see *Sù Wèn* 《素問》 8 and 69), the expression is, however, also used in the sense of the outward radiance of cosmological or personal essence as the reflection of an enlightened ruler's or sage's embodiment of the Dào. Therefore I have intentionally left it literal and less specific so that readers can interpret the phrase in as narrow or broad a meaning as they like. I am indebted to the participants of the "Scholars of Chinese Medicine" Facebook page, especially Leo Lok, for helping me shine our own light on this difficult term.

5. According to the *Míng Yī Bié Lù* 《名醫別錄》 ("Separate Records by Famous Physicians," compiled by Táo Hóngjǐng 陶弘景 in the early fifth century. See p. xl in the Preface),

the different types of ganoderma are distinguished by their area of origin: "Red ganoderma grows on Huòshān, black ganoderma on Héngshān, green-blue ganoderma on Tàishān, white ganoderma on Huáshān, yellow ganoderma on Hāoshān, and purple ganoderma in high locations in China." The precise identity of these mushrooms continues to be subject to scholarly debate and scientific research. In contemporary practice, *Ganoderma lucidum* or *japonicum* are used.

6. This is the same plant, alternately referred to as *Saposhnikovia divaricata*, *Ledebouriella divaricata*, or *Ledebouriella seseloides*.

7. Also called *Hylotelephium erythrostictum*.

8. *Dùhéng* is a more common medicinal ingredient, identified as *Asarum forbesii* (Southern asarum). It is important to note, however, that even early pharmaceutical literature does sometimes distinguish between the two substances.

9. Note that the term "demon inspector" has already been mentioned as an alternate name for *chìjiàn* (page 71).

10. The more common modern name for this medicinal is *ròuguì* 肉桂, whether as twigs (*guìzhī* 桂枝) or core (*guìxīn* 桂心).

11. This term most likely refers to the high-grade variety of cinnamon, which is now more commonly known as *guānguì* 官桂 ("officials' cinnamon").

12. While both the bark of the root and the fruit are used in Chinese medicine, the entry here has historically been identified with the medicinal that is now called *gǒuqǐgēn* 枸杞根 ("wolfsberry root") or *dìgǔpí* 地骨皮 ("skin of earth bone"). In contemporary practice, the berries are used more commonly and often come from *Lycium barbarum* instead.

13. The phrase *rè zhòng* 熱中 is a technical term referring to a disease that is described in the *Sù Wèn* as related to wind strike and resulting in yellowing of the eyes. It is not identical with 中熱 ("heat strike").

14. Now more commonly known as *bǎizǐrén* 柏子仁.

15. Beginning with Táo Hóngjǐng 陶弘景, this line has historically been interpreted as referring to *mǔjīngzǐ* 牡荊子, fruit of *Vitex negundo L. var. cannabifolia* (hemp-leaved vitex fruit).

16. All of these species used to be subsumed under the genus *Acanthopanax*, under which it is still commonly known in Chinese medicine circles, but modern taxonomy has adopted *Eleutherococcus* as the official name.

17. More commonly called *ruírén* 蕤仁 in contemporary Chinese medicine.

18. In contemporary practice, *fùpén* is identified with *Rubus chingii*, while *pénglěi* is treated as a different plant, identified with *Rubus tephrodus*. Throughout Chinese history, however, these two species have often been used interchangeably.

19. Translated literally, the Chinese name simply means "bitter greens." It is likely that many other kinds of "bitter greens," depending on historical and regional differences, fall into this rather large and nondescript category. My identification with *Solanchus oleraceus* is based on the information from the *Zhōngyào Dà Cídiǎn* 《中藥大辭典》 ("Great Dictionary of Chinese Medicinals," 1982 edition).

20. While here given as an alternate name and therefore substitute for *xiāoshí*, the two substances are distinguished in other texts.

21. It is also possible to read the term *dōnghǎi* 東海 (lit. "eastern sea") as a reference to the far eastern regions of China in general, similar to the meaning of 南海 (lit. "southern sea"), which in this text refers to the far south, such as in the entry for *mǔguì* 牧桂 (page 110).

22. In contemporary Chinese medicine practice and in most historical writings, *yǔyúliáng* and *tàiyīyúliáng* are identified as the same substance. I am here following the literal text and structure of the earliest edition of my source text, as reconstructed in the critical edition by the contemporary medical historian Mǎ Jìxìng. According to the *Běncǎo Gāng Mù* 《本草綱目》, ("Systematic Materia Medica," published in 1596, by Lǐ Shízhēn 李時珍) the only difference between these two substances is their place of origin.

23. While *zǐshíyīng* is usually identified with fluorite in contemporary Chinese medicine literature, fluorite is not a variety of quartz, as the Chinese name "purple quartz" implies. Amethyst, on the other hand, fits this description perfectly since it is precisely the purple variety of quartz.

24. In contemporary Chinese medicine, this medicinal is identified with halloysite.

25. According to the *Táng Běncǎo* 《唐本草》 ("Táng Materia Medica," also known as *Xīn Xiū Běncǎo* 《新修本草》, published 657-659 by Sū Jìng 蘇敬), "What Táo Hóngjǐng refers to as white azurite is what we now call *kōngqīng* ("hollow azurite"), round like a pearl made of iron, whitish and without a hollow center. When you grind it up, the color is whitish like light jade, which is the reason why it is also called *bìqīng* 碧青. It is not used for paint pigment…"

26. According to the *Běncǎo Gāng Mù*, *biǎnqīng* is the variety of azurite used by painters as pigment, also known as *dàqīng* 大青 ("great green-blue").

27. I am grateful to Leo Lok for pointing out that this is the only substance where the notion of "facilitating the breakthrough of spirit illumination" (通神 or 通神明) is not listed as an effect of long-term consumption for the purpose of alchemical transformation (久服). As such, this phrase needs to be regarded differently here from the context of practices aimed at transcendence (神仙). Instead, it is found alongside terms like "killing toxin" (殺毒), "warding off bad luck" (辟不祥), and "killing demons" (殺鬼). In other words, it belongs to the category of *zhù yóu* 祝由, exorcistic treatments.

28. Chinese scholars have disagreed over the meaning of this phrase for many centuries, with interpretations ranging from mysterious eggs laid by roosters (lacking the yolk) to the intestines and other pouch-like areas in roosters.

中藥

MIDDLE MEDICINALS

NOTES

1. This medicinal is known more commonly in contemporary materia medica texts as *cāngěrzǐ* 蒼耳子.

2. Other varieties of *Pueraria*, such as *P. edulis, thomsonii, omeiensis*, or *phaseoloides*, are used locally.

3. The root is now more commonly known as *tiānhuāfěn* 天花粉 ("Heaven Flower Powder").

4. The name for this medicinal can also be pronounced as lǐshí but must not be confused with the medicinal with that name lǐshí ("fibrous gypsum" on page 288).

5. Also known as *mǎlìn* 馬藺.

6. This four-character expression is an interesting variation on the more common phrase *duò tāi* 墮胎, the customary term for abortifacients. Similar to some of the other actions of this medicinal, the phrase here means that *qúmài* has the power to disperse or disintegrate a congealing fetus by interrupting and reversing the natural action of progressive binding and hardening, similar to its effect of bursting welling-abscesses or breaking up blocked blood.

7. Sometimes also *Lilium brownii*.

8. In contemporary TCM literature, the plant is usually referred to as *báimáo* 白茅.

9. I have been unable to arrive at a positive identification for this plant. While *zǐshēn* is often equated with *Salvia chinensis* or *Rubia yunnanensis*, it is not listed in the *Zhōngyào Dà Cídiǎn* 《中藥大辭典》. Its alternate name *mǔméng* is there identified with *Paris tetraphylla* (more commonly known as *wángsūn* 王孫). Dr. Eugene Anderson, however, equates *mǔméng* with *Polyganum bistorta*.

10. Rather than imposing my tentative interpretation, I have kept my translation literal, to let the reader make up their own mind about this interesting phrase. While often associated with the joints, especially in the compound *guānjié* 關節, 關 literally means barred door and from there by extension "barrier," "mountain pass," "critical juncture," or just "closing" in general. Most likely, the phrase refers here to the joints. I am indebted to Leo Lok for reminding me that the term *jī guān* 機關 is used in the *Huáng Dì Nèi Jīng* 《黃帝內經》 ("Yellow Emperor's Inner Classic," comp. in the Hàn period) to refer to either the joints of the neck and lumbus (*Sù Wèn* 45: "On Reversal") or the shoulders, elbows, hips and knees (*Líng Shū* 71: "Evil Intrusion").

11. The identity of this herb was already unclear by the time of Táo Hóngjǐng, who comments that people no longer use

it and that its medicinal effect is similar to *báihuāténg* 白花藤 (*Clematis maximowicziana*).

12. The hot qì that is discharged during sweating.

13. Locally also *Stephania tetranda* 漢防己 or *Cocculus trilobus* 木防己.

14. Also known as *Justicia procumbens*.

15. The botanical identification of this herb is highly problematic. Táo Hóngjǐng already mentions that it was no longer in use at his time but that there was a formula called Gùhuó Wán 固活丸 (Gùhuó Pills) that used the herb commonly known as *yěgé* 野葛 "wild kudzu." This substance is usually identified as the whole plant of *Gelsemium elegans* (see *gōuwěn* 鈎吻 (*Gelsemium elegans*) on page 323, which gives *yěgé* as an alternate name). Nevertheless, equating *gūhuó* with *gùhuó* is questionable at best, as other commentaries point out. It is furthermore important to note that Táo Hóngjǐng specifically stated that this kind of *dōngkuízǐ* must not be equated with the normal substance referred to by the same name, which is identified with *Malva verticillata*.

16. The identity of this herb is unknown. Some editions of the Divine Farmer's Classic have "root and fruit" after the name, and some list it in the lower category of medicinals.

According to Táo Hóngjǐng, this medicinal was no longer in use at his time.

17. As in the previous entry, the identity of this herb is unknown and it had already fallen out of use in Táo Hóngjǐng's times.

18. In the *Běncǎo Gāng Mù*, Lǐ Shízhēn lists this medicinal under *liánqiáo* 連翹 (fruit of *Forsythia suspensa*), in which case we could simply identify this entry here as "forsythia root." I am not certain, however, that this term here does in fact refer to the root of *liánqiáo*.

19. Due to the grammatical vagaries of classical Chinese, it is impossible to say whether *yīn jīng* 陰精 means "yīn essence" (i.e., a particular type of essence that is associated with yīn) or "yīn and essence." I have tried to replicate this semantic openness by adding the square brackets around "and."

20. While the text does not specify which part of the plant to use medicinally, and the root tends to be referred to more specifically as *xuāncǎogēn* 萱草根 "orange day-lily root," I follow Táo Hóngjǐng and the commentary tradition in accepting that this entry refers to the root here instead of the flower or whole plant.

21. This character should refer to *shízhūyú* 食茱萸, Zanthoxylum ailanthoides, but is also used to refer to *shānzhūyú* 山茱萸, Cornus officinalis.

22. I follow the commentary tradition and read yáng 陽 here as a textual error for *yáng* 瘍. Another possibility suggested by some commentators would be to read the character as a mistake for *shāng* 傷, "damage."

23. Unfortunately, it is unclear to me how this substance differs from the "mulberry wood ear" described in the previous sentence. Pronounced *nòu*, the character 檽 refers to a type of tree, but pronounced *ruǎn* it is used as a synonym for *mùěr* 木耳 "wood ear" in general.

24. Inch Whiteworm is a technical term that is most likely referring to tapeworm infestation.

25. Both *língtiáo* and *zǐwěi* are less common names for the medicinals that is now usually referred to as *língxiāohuā* 凌霄花.

26. Depending on context, the term *diān* 癲, which I have here translated as "Epilepsy," can have two different meanings in classical Chinese medical literature and is therefore alternately translated as "Epilepsy" or "Mania." Usually written in the compound *diānxián* 癲癇, it refers to Epilepsy;

in the compounds *diānkuáng* 癲狂 or *fēngdiān* 瘋癲, it refers to a particular type of insanity that is associated with yīn. As a third alternative, some later editions of this text and therefore also some commentators read 癲 as a textual error for *lài* 癩, meaning "leprosy." I have decided to interpret it as Epilepsy for three reasons: first because of the etymology of the character includes the concept of jolting or toppling (*diān* 顛), second because some early editions actually have the character 顛 instead of 癲, and third because the compound 癲疾, as written above, is clearly defined as referring to epileptic fits in such important early classics as the *Líng Shū* (see *Líng Shū* 22). Arguably, the interpretation as "leprosy" is also possible given its context here after "malign wind." Another common name for leprosy in classical sources is, after all, "hemp/numbness wind" (*máfēng* 麻風).

27. While the term *fēngshuǐ* 風水 is well-known in English in the context of such fields as architecture and interior design, when it is often somewhat inaccurately translated as "geomancy," its technical meaning in medical literature is a bit more complex. As outlined in the *Jīn Guì Yào Lüè* chapter on "Water Qì," Wind Water refers to the internal presence of water qì that is complicated by externally contracted wind evil. Manifesting in aversion to wind and sore bones and joints in addition to puffy swelling especially in the face and upper body, it is an exterior condition.

28. Based on several later editions, I assume that the term *héhuān* here refers specifically to the bark, more commonly referred to as *héhuānpí* 合歡皮 in contemporary literature.

29. In contemporary medicinal literature, this substance is more commonly referred to as *liǎngmiànzhēn* 兩面針 or as *rùdìjīnniú* 入地金牛.

30. Identity unknown.

31. Also known as "flowering apricot." This substance is often identified incorrectly in English literature as "plum."

32. In later medical literature, "killing grain" is seen as a pathology related to excess heat in the stomach that is accelerating the stomach's digestive function and thereby preventing the appropriate absorption of nutrients. Here, however, the expression must be referring to an intended medicinal effect of *shuǐsū*, most likely related to longevity practices aimed at making the body lighter and connecting it to heaven instead of weighing it down towards the earth. As such, it might have prepared the adept's body for the eventual practice of *bì gǔ* 避穀, of eliminating grain from one's diet altogether and gradually transitioning the body to subsisting on nothing but qì and some medicinal substances.

33. According to Leo Lok, the expression 多熱令人煩 should here be read quite differently as "[eaten] in excess, causes heat and vexation." Besides the fact that *shǔmǐ*, when eaten in large quantities, is indeed hard to digest, Lok suggests that the character 熱 "heat" could here be a mistake for the character 食 "to eat". Based on the fact that *shǔmǐ* is said in the *Míng Yī Bié Lù* to "eliminate heat and stop vexation and thirst" 除熱止煩渴, I am not convinced by this line of reasoning but offer it here as a plausible alternative reading.

34. I have translated this term literally because I have been unable to identify it positively with a particular plant. The term refers to a cinnabar-colored variety of broomcorn millet that was primarily used for ancestral sacrifices.

35. The identification of *máfén* is surprisingly tricky. While it is usually translated as "hemp seed" and often equated in contemporary sources with the term *mázǐ* 麻子 "hemp seed," the listing and separate description of *mázǐ* below must mean that *máfén* refers to a different part of the plant. Based on early descriptions, it appears to refer to the full fruit, i.e., the inner seed as well as the pericarp.

36. As in the case of *yǔyúliáng* on page 153, it is also possible to read the compound *dōnghǎi* 東海 "eastern sea" as a general reference to the far eastern regions of China.

37. According to a lengthy commentary in the *Běncǎo Jīng Jí Zhù* 《神農本草經輯注》 ("Edited and Annotated Divine Farmer's Classic of Materia Medica," edited by Mǎ Jīxìng and published in 1995), the expression *suānxiāo* 酸痟 is more likely to refer to soreness and pain that comes from debilitation due to "paring down" or "whittling away" (削) of the body. See pp. 302-303 in said reference. The earliest Chinese dictionary from the Hàn dynasty, the *Shuō Wén Jiě Zì* 《說文解字》 ("Explaining Graphs and Analyzing Characters," 2nd c. CE), however, defines 痟 as 酸痟頭痛 "a sore and debilitating headache."

38. This term tends to be used specifically for women's conditions of vaginal hemorrhaging. Given that it is here followed by another common gynecological term (*lòu* 漏 "spotting" followed by mentioning of the uterus, it is clear to me that the first few symptoms listed here refer to women's disorders.

39. Unfortunately, I have been unable to positively confirm the identity of this substance and the following one. While they appear to be some type of stalactite, their relationship to *shízhōngrǔ* 石鐘乳 (page 146) was already unclear during Táo Hóngjǐng's times. In discussing three medicinals derived from stalactites, he describes *kǒnggōngniè* as "coiled deposits formed over long periods of time by fluids dripping from the roof of caves." He also calls them "*zhōngrǔ*

beds" (鍾乳床), or in other words the "base" of *zhōngrǔ* (the "nipple" of the formations). In contrast, and second-best, are "smaller pairs" (小雙) of stalactites, which he identifies with *yīnniè*. The part of the stalactite that is light in weight and formed by further dripping from this *yīnniè* is what is called *zhōngrǔ*. Disagreeing with this differentiation, Lǐ Shízhēn quotes Sū Gōng as offering the following theory: "*Yīn*[*niè*] is like the root of the breast, *kǒnggōng* like the actual breast itself, and *zhōngrǔ* like the nipple." See, for example, the entry on *zhōngrǔ* 鍾乳 in the *Běncǎo Gāng Mù*.

40. This last line has caused much discussion and confusion over the centuries among commentators and been explained in many different ways. The key difference between readings is whether the term *shén* 神 is interpreted as referring to the "spirit(s)" of the person ingesting the medicinal or whether it should be interpreted adverbially, so that *shénhuà* 神化 should be read as a verbal compound meaning "divine transformation." Related to this and following the first reading, *shén* can function as the object of *huán* 還, which is then understood in the sense of "returning" or "bringing home." Otherwise it can be interpreted as "revert" or "turn around," thus referring not to bringing home the *shén*, but to the substance itself returning to its original state. In classical Chinese medicine, the hair on the head is the "remainder of blood" 血餘, and is therefore known for its association with and effect on the blood, most notably by stopping bleeding.

"Divine transformation" could thus refer to the fact that hair is formed from the "left-overs" of blood, is prepared in alchemical and medical practice by ashing to be ingested as a medicinal, and then returns into the body to once again feed the blood. Either way, it is clearly associated with restoring the free and healthy flow of blood in the body, which when obstructed or blocked has dramatic effects on the *shén*, such as pediatric Seizures or adult tetany. Lastly, it may be significant that the term used for "transform" here, *huà* 化, is one of two terms used to express change in classical medical literature, the other being *biàn* 變. While *biàn* describes change in the sense of alterations or fluctuations (such as day and night, yīn and yáng, the recurring and never-ending cycle of the seasons, etc.), *huà* refers to a more drastic, irreversible, substantive type of change that is perhaps best translated as "metamorphosis," an actual transcendence of the form, such as the change from the pupa to the butterfly. Both *huán* and *huà* are used in alchemical literature but in what ways these specific technical connotations play into the reading of this particular phrase here is unclear to me.

41. In other words, it boosts fertility.

42. In other animals, the term *xuántí* 懸蹄 refers to the dewclaw. Since horses don't have dewclaws, my best guess is that it refers to the soft inner part of the hoof, specifically the frog.

下藥

Lower Medicinals

Notes

1. Sometimes also *Aconitum kusnezoffii*, so-called "wild aconite."

2. *Hóu bì yān tòng* 喉痹咽痛: Because of my intention with this book to be as true to the original as possible, I have chosen to translate this four-character expression literally here, instead of in the broader sense of "*Bì* Impediment and pain in the throat."

3. This medicinal is more commonly known today as *chángshān* 常山.

4. See page 320 for *cǎohāo*.

5. According to Lǐ Shízhēn, who quotes Sū Gōng, this mushroom "now comes from Bóhǎi 渤海 (between Liaodong and Shandong peninsulas) and grows naturally in salty ground among reeds in marshes. It is not formed from stork's manure. The mushroom is white, light, hollow, looks the same on the inside and outside surfaces, and is different from normal mushrooms. It is effective in treating roundworm." This information contradicts Táo Hóngjǐng's 陶弘景 theory that the mushroom does indeed grow out of stork manure. I have been unable to positively identify this plant.

6. Often adulterated with *Knoxia valerianoides*.

7. Other genera include *Woodwardia unigemmata* (chain fern), *Osmunda japonica* (royal fern), *Brainia insignis,* and *Matteuccia struthiopteris* (ostrich fern).

8. The positive identification of this substance is unfortunately impossible. Bernard Read identifies it as *Potentilla cryptotaenia* in his Chinese Medicinal Plants from the Pen Ts'ao Kang Mu (first published in 1900), while Mǎ Jīxìng offers *Agrimonia pilosa*, agrimony root, as an alternative in his *Mǎwángduī gǔ yīshū kǎoshì* 《馬王堆古醫書考釋》 ("Philological Investigation of the Ancient Medical Texts from Mawangdui," published in 1992). *Agrimonia pilosa* is also the plant identified with *lángyá*, its alternate name, in the *Zhōnghuá Běncǎo* 《中華本草》 ("Chinese Materia Medica," published in 1999), but the evidence is too tentative to draw any firm conclusions.

9. Regionally also *Euphorbia fisheriana* or *ebiacteolata*, which can then be referred to as *báilángdú* 白狼毒 "white *lángdú*."

10. Usually, the term *yángtáo* 羊桃 "sheep/goat peach" is identified with starfruit (*Averrhoa carambola*), which is correctly written as *yángtáo* 陽桃 "yáng peach." Nevertheless, the present context in the lowest category of medicinals and its description as toxic and hence with strong medicinal efficacy makes this identification here implausible. The term is more likely used here to refer to *Actinidia chinensis* (Chinese

gooseberry), which is more commonly called *míhóutáo* "Rhesus macaque peach," but can also be called *yángtáo*, written as either 羊桃 or 陽桃. In the *Zhōngyào Dà Cídiǎn*, the fruit is described as resolving heat, disinhibiting urination, and treating strangury, among other actions, which overlaps somewhat with the actions described above for the root. Note that *Actinidia deliciosa*, the famous kiwifruit commonly believed to be native to New Zealand, is either identical with or a cultivated form of *Actinidia chinensis*. The root of *Actinidia chinensis* is described in the *Zhōngyào Dà Cídiǎn* as cool and slightly toxic and as indicated for "clearing heat, disinhibiting urination, enlivening blood, and dispersing swelling. It treats liver inflammation, water swelling, injuries from physical trauma, wind-damp joint pain, turbid strangury, …"

11. Plant of unknown identity, most likely closely related or identical with *luómó* 蘿藦, *Metaplexis japonica*. Already during Táo Hóngjǐng's time, the identity of this plant was debated. Táo cites three theories: 1. that it is identical with *luómó*; 2. that it is close relative of *luómó*; and 3. that it is the name for the root of *shéhǎn*. Táo himself finds the third option unlikely both because of the morphological description of the plant and because of the difference in natural habitat and plant parts used. Moreover, the offensive odor associated with *nǚqīng* suggests a close relation with other plants in the Milkweed family, such as carrion flower (*Stapelia* or

Huernia). It is perhaps for this reason that the *Zhōngyào Dà Cídiǎn* lists it as a synonym for *jīshǐténg* 雞屎藤 (*Paedaria scandens*).

12. Note that this identification is based on the fact that *xúchángqīng* is given as an alternate name and that substance is commonly identified with *Cynanchum paniculatum*. Nevertheless, *xúchāngqíng* is described as a separate substance in "xúchángqīng" on page 103.

13. For an explanation of *kuángyáng* 狂昜 as my translation of *zhù yì* 注易, see Glossary entry on Mania. I have chosen to follow the commentary tradition and the version of the text in some editions and therefore read *zhù* 注 as *kuáng* 狂 "Mania" and *yì* 易 as *yáng* 昜, which is an older version of 陽. This reading fits nicely with the following symptoms.

14. Substance derived from an herb of unknown origin. Táo Hóngjǐng offers two alternate names: *lílóu* 離婁 and *juéjù* 掘据. In the *Grand Ricci* dictionary (originally called Le Grand Dictionnaire de la Langue Chinoise and published in 2001, comp. by Jean Lefeuvre et al.), *lílóu* is defined as *Euphorbia lathyris*, but I have not been able to find any information on *juéjù*.

15. This identification is based on the fact that it is offered as an alternative name for *dàyèjiīnhuācǎo* 大葉金花草 in the

Zhōngyào Dà Cídiǎn. The same plant is also known as *Sphenomeric chinensis* or "lace fern."

16. I follow most commentators and read *diān* 癲 here in the sense of *diān* 巔 "head" or "vertex." The two characters are frequently used interchangeably, and since *diān* 癲 is more common, it is often used as a substitute for and in the sense of 巔. The combination of 巔 with the character *jí* 疾 "disease," particularly one of a racing, urgent character, as a compound can mean "urgent conditions of the vertex" but is in most cases used as the standard technical term to mean Epilepsy. The alternate meaning of 癲 as a yīn-type of dementia, translated by Wiseman quite appropriately as "withdrawal," seems less likely here in the compound phrase 癲疾.

17. .It is unclear here whether treating "cow lice and small worms" refers to the medicinal efficacy of *niúbiǎn* in treating a variety of lice called "cow lice" and small worms in humans, or whether this phrase here means that *niúbiǎn* can be used as a treatment for lice and worms in livestock. In contemporary literature, the term *niúshī* 牛蝨 "cow louse" refers specifically to *Haematopinus eurysternus* or "ungulate louse."

18. Some editions have *lúfù* 鹿腹 "deer abdomen" or *lútóu* 鹿頭 "deer head" instead.

19. It is unclear to me whether the expression *huǒchuáng* 火瘡 "fire sores/wounds" refers to wounds that the patient has sustained as the result of exposure to fire, i.e. burns, or whether this is a reference to a type of skin disorder that is associated with fire among the Five Agents. I tend to read it in the first sense, only because I have not seen skin conditions, generally seen as a manifestation of pathogenic internal heat, categorized by reference to one of the Five Agents elsewhere. Of course physical external fire as an etiological agent is never far from its understanding as an internal factor. Ultimately, it may simply be the wrong question to ask whether "fire" here is an internal or external agent because they should both be treated identically. As such, they are of course associated with the color red.

20. According to the note in *Běncǎo Jīng Jí Zhù*, this term describes an acute inflammatory condition characterized by redness and swelling in the skin. Unfortunately, no information is given about the origin of this explanation.

21. Possibly also *Zanthoxylum simulans* or *schinifolium*. *Shǔjiāo* is often given as an alternate name for *huājiāo* 花椒, *qínjiāo* 秦椒, or *chuānjiāo* 川椒, but these substances may or may not be identical. Sūn Sīmiǎo, for example, apparently distinguishes between *shǔjiāo* 蜀椒 and *qínjiāo* 秦椒. Shǔ 蜀 and Qín 秦 were two neighboring states in the Warring States period, both located in the far west. The state of Shǔ, located to the

south of Qín in what is now the western Sìchuān basin, was conquered and absorbed by the state of Qín in 316 BCE. So it is possible that the two names *shǔjiāo* and *qínjiāo* refer to two closely related varieties of *Zanthoxylum* growing in the southern (Shǔ) and northern (Qín) part of China's far west, or that the two names refer to the same plant, with *shǔjiāo* "Shǔ peppercorn" simply being an older term that was replaced after the victory of Qín with *qínjiāo* "Qín peppercorn," and has now been replaced yet again with *chuānjiāo* 川椒 "Sìchuān peppercorn" for the modern name of the province that covers that region.

22. My addition of this word here is based on a version of the text that includes the characters 「中寒冷去」 between 皮膚 and 死肌. Several other editions lack the character 死 "dead" and have 溫 "warm" instead of 濕 "damp."

23. In most contexts, the character *liàn* 楝 refers to a more common species, *Melia azedarach*, known in English as white cedar, chinaberry tree, or Persian lilac. In contemporary TCM literature, this medicinal is more commonly known as *chuānliànzǐ* 川楝子.

24. Prior to its reclassification in 1995, it was known as *Polyporus mylittae* and is often still identified as such. As yet another Latin name, the same mushroom is also sometimes referred to as *Omphalia lapidescens*.

25. Strictly speaking, *zhàngfū* 丈夫 means "husband," but especially in medical literature it is commonly used to refer to adult men.

26. One of the earliest Chinese dictionaries called the *Guǎng Yǎ* 《廣雅》 ("Expanded Ěryǎ," compiled in the early third century CE by Zhāng Yī 張揖), a third century CE dictionary, offers *yàoshí* 藥實 as an alternate name for *bèifù* 貝父 (*Fritillaria cirrhosa* and related species) but this identification is not repeated or confirmed in materia medica literature.

27. My identification is based on an eleventh century commentary to a Táng dynasty poem that explains *huánghuán* as an alternate name for *zhūténg* 朱藤, which is more commonly known as *zǐténg* 紫藤. The other names offered in the text above fail to shed any more light on the problem of identifying this substance.

28. More commonly known as *jīngjiè* 荊芥.

29. According to the *Zhōngyào Dà Cídiǎn*, to process this substance further, the dried bean sprouts are simmered with the stem and leaves of *Lopatherum gracile* and the pith from *Juncus effusus* until the fluid has evaporated, and then sundried again.

30. This generic term may refer to both *Vigna angularis* (adzuki bean) and *V. umbellata*, previously known as *Phaseolus calcaratus* (ricebean).

31. This identification is questionable at best. As already mentioned by Táo Hóngjǐng, the same name is used in later materia medica literature to refer to a completely different medicinal: the stalk and leaf (or root, when specified as such) of *Premna microphylla* (*dòufǔmù* 豆腐木). Given the location here in the section on foodstuff, I find the literal meaning of "bean flower" more likely, at least for the time of the *Shén Nóng Běncǎo Jīng*.

32. "Five Weapons" is a stock phrase to refer to all the different weapons current during the classical age. In the earliest sources, such as the *Zhōu Lǐ* 《周禮》 ("Rites of Zhōu," first evidence from the 2nd c. BCE but edited by Liú Xīn 劉歆 during the mid Hàn dynasty), these are listed as: *gē* 戈 "halberd or dagger-ax," *shū* 殳 "bamboo lance," *jǐ* 戟 "two-pronged pole-weapon," *qiúmáo* 酋矛 "short-handled spear," and *yímáo* 夷矛 "long lance." Other versions include swords, bows and arrows, etc., reflecting the development of weaponry over time. The statement here that realgar prevails over the Five Weapons presumable means that it is a substance that makes you impregnable by weapons. Whether this effect is achieved by taking the substance internally or by

carrying it on your body, as suggested by the commentary in the *Běncǎo Jīng Jí Zhù*, is unclear.

33. See entry 6 on page 454.

34. The identity of this substance is unknown. Táo Hóngjǐng already commented that it was no longer used at his time and that he did not know anything about it.

35. This line has been stumping commentators for millennia apparently. Táo Hóngjǐng explains that *huángdān* 黃丹 "yellow cinnabar," an alternate name for *qiāndān*, is formed by heating lead 鉛, and that this substance must be rubbed on cauldrons that are used to prepare elixirs. In his reading, this line should mean that "Nine Radiance Elixir can only be produced in a cauldron made with this substance, and there is no other method." There is also the possibility that the standard identification of *qiāndān* as "minium" might be mistaken, and that the text is really talking about "litharge," a natural mineral form of lead oxide that can also be produced as a by-product when heating lead to 600°C. At least some of the commentators distinguish between 黃丹 *huángdān* and 鉛丹 *qiāndān*. Another alternate name for the substance is 鉛華 "lead bloom." According to Nathan Sivin (*Chinese Alchemy: Preliminary Studies*, p. 149), the "Nine-Fold-Radiance" is identified as massicot, another lead oxide that

is yellow and can occur both naturally and as a by-product of lead oxidation.

36. According to one historical commentary cited in the *Běncǎo Jīng Jí Zhù*, "lurking intestines" is an ancient disease term that refers to inauspicious concretions in the interior.

37. I have translated this term literally to retain the ambivalent meaning of the Chinese original. "Interrupted pregnancy" could refer either to a problem with repeated miscarriages or to an interruption in the ability to get pregnant in the first place.

38. In the *Běncǎo Gāng Mù*, this substance is, as here, listed in the section on "Rocks," as opposed to *shíjiǎn* 石鹼 "stone salt," which is identified with *huījiǎn* 灰鹼 "ash salt" and listed in the section on "Soils." Cited there, Wú Pǔ 吳普 stresses that this substance is the salt from bittern (*lǔshuǐ* 鹵水), not the salt from salt-rich soil. Lǐ Shízhēn explains that *lǔxián* refers to the hard mineral deposit that settles on the bottom of the "bitter water" that is the by-product when halite (common salt) is evaporated from seawater or brines.

『凡鹽未經滴去苦水,則不堪食,苦水即鹵水也。鹵水之下,澄鹽凝結如石者,即鹵鹼也。丹溪所謂石鹼者,乃灰鹼也,見土類。吳普《本草》謂鹵鹼一名鹵鹽者,指鹵水之鹽,非鹵地之鹽也,不妨同名。』

39. Also identified as azurite, spinel, or Balas ruby in various modern sources, the more common name for malachite is *lùqīng* 綠青. Alternately, the same term is used later to refer to the skeleton of *Acropora pulchra*, a type of stony coral that is pink but turns grey or black when taken out of the ocean. This usage does not fit here, however, given the listing under "Rocks" (i.e., minerals), its associated medicinal actions, and the fact that the early commentary in the *Míng Yī Bié Lù* describe it as coming from the area of Shǔ 蜀, i.e., modern Sichuan.

40. The *Běncǎo Gāng Mù* states that this substance is toxic.

41. My reading of what could literally be "hemorrhoid worms" or "Hemorrhoids and worms" as "hemorrhoid[-causing] worms" is based on a line in the *Zhū Bìng Yuán Hòu Lùn*: "Pinworms are extremely tiny, like maggots in vegetables. They dwell in the intestines and, when profuse, cause Hemorrhoids."

42. According to Táo Hóngjǐng, "winter ash" refers to the yellow ash that was used in his time to wash clothes, produced by burning the stalks and leaves from different herbs like artemisia and chenopodium. The most powerful ashes were supposedly produced by burning Amur silver grass (*dí* 荻, *Miscanthus sacchariflorus*). According to Lǐ Shízhēn, on the other hand, "winter ash" refers literally to the ashes

that were produced by burning firewood in the kitchen stove during the winter months and does not have to be derived from burning specific herbs. Lǐ also mentions that his contemporaries use the soda from the ashes for washing clothes, lightening skin, treating malign sores, and for dying with indigo.

43. The standard interpretation of this term is horse, cattle, sheep and goat, chickens, dogs, and pigs. According to the commentary in the *Běncǎo Jīng Jí Zhù*, "hair" refers to the skin and fur, "hoof" to the entire foot, and "nail" to the claws and nails.

44. In later editions, the information on rhinoceros horn is listed as a separate entry, which does make sense since rhinoceroses are not generally regarded as livestock.

45. The section on "Epidemic Pestilences" in volume 10 of the *Zhū Bìng Yuán Hòu Lùn* contains an essay on *zhàng* qì 瘴氣, which I translate as "Southern miasmic qì." Here, Cháo Yuánfāng explains that *zhàng* in the area south of the "Five Ridges" (i.e., Guangdong and Guangxi) is like Cold Damage in the area to the north. Because of the warm climate in the south, the plants do not drop their leaves and the insects do not go underground during the time of Tàiyīn. Instead, this warmth produces all sorts of toxins. Specifically, the "miasm of green grass" (青草瘴) prevails from the second month of

spring to the second month of summer, and the "miasm of yellow awns" from the last month of summer to the first month of winter. And while people in the South still fall ill with Cold Damage, their symptoms manifest differently and they must be treated differently, with restricted use of hot medicinals and no "reckless attack with hot decoctions and moxibustion." If treated too aggressively, the illness can advance into the interior and develop into jaundice, which can over time develop further into "corpse jaundice." This is a condition that the locals do not need to be treated for because they are exposed to the miasmic qì on a continuous basis. Visitors from the North, however, require careful deliberation to be rescued. Specifically, the physician must distinguish between yīn and yáng contractions and consequently attack the patient's inside or outside respectively.

46. I.e., *Gelsemium elegans*, a highly toxic plant described on page 323.

47. The *zhēn* bird is either a mythological creature dreaded because of its poisonous feathers or the serpent eagle (Spilornis cheela), a raptor famous for its appetite for poisonous insects. In either case, the feathers dipped in wine were believed to kill the person purposely or inadvertently exposed to them.

48. I disagree with the punctuation of most modern editions here and interpret *nán hǎi* 南海 (lit., "south sea") not as the South China Sea but in the sense of "far south." It is clearly used in this sense in other places in the *Shén Nóng Běncǎo Jīng*, such as when describing the place of origin of stalactites (page 290). Standard modern editions place a *dùnhào* 頓號 (a kind of Chinese comma, used to mark off items in a list) between *nánhǎi* and *chízé* (南海、池澤), which would be translated as "in the South China Sea and in ponds and marshes." In addition to precedence, my other argument for my reading is that Reeve's turtle is a semiaquatic freshwater turtle that lives in marshes and shallow ponds and would not survive in the South China Sea.

49. Some historical editions have *shànyú* 鱓魚 (according to the *Grand Ricci* dictionary identified as *Monopterus albus*, Asian swamp eel) instead. This identification makes no sense, however, since swamp eels don't have shells to be turned into a medicinal substance. In the *Shuō Wén Jiě Zì* dictionary, *shànyú* is explained as the name of a fish with a skin that can be turned into a drum. According to the *Ěr Yǎ*, *shànyú* has two meanings: one describes a snake-like fish, clearly a reference to the Asian swamp eel, with which it is identified nowadays, and second, to a shark, *Mustelus manazo* (starspotted smooth-hound, a type of houndshark). Under this second definition, it does in fact give 鮀魚 as an alternate name. Nevertheless, as the *Běncǎo Jīng Jí Zhù* points

out, none of these options make sense here since we are looking for an aquatic animal with a hard carapace (*jiǎ* 甲).

50. Locally also *P. olivaceus* or *Parapolyhia vara*. This substance is often referred to in English as "hornet's nest" but hornet refers to the genus *Vespula*, which is considerably more toxic than the paper wasp.

51. According to Táo Hóngjǐng's commentary, this phrase means that crab has the effect of neutralizing the toxicity of lacquer by "transforming it into water" 化漆為水.

52. Again, Táo's commentary is helpful and clarifies that the smoke from burning crab can be used for rodent control because it causes all the rodents to appear.

53. In modern times as a medicinal ingredient, this substance tends to be derived from *Elaphe taeniurus*, *E. carinata*, and similar species in the Rat Snake genus.

54. No commentator gives any explanation about this line, so I have simply translated it literally and leave it to the reader's discretion to figure out what this means. My sense is that it does not refer to killing the hedgehog by boiling it in liquor but that the medicinal, when decocted in liquor instead of in plain water, "kills" all the conditions listed above, in the sense of subduing them.

55. See Note 21 above and the Glossary entry on Mania for the meaning of *kuángyáng* 狂易.

56. The phrase 好色 is commonly read as *hào sè* and interpreted as "to love sex." In the present context, however, I am quite certain that *sè* 色 refers not to sexual intercourse but to the more literal meaning "color," or here specifically the complexion of the body, as in the compound *yán sè* 顏色 "facial complexion." The expression *hǎo yán sè* 好顏色, which I translate as "beautifies the facial complexion," is found numerous times in the *Shén Nóng Běncǎo Jīng*.

57. At first glance, it might be tempting to read *shénjīng* 神精 here as a textual error for *shénmíng* 神明, given how often the action of "facilitating the breakthrough of spirit illumination" occurs as a set phrase in the *Shén Nóng Běncǎo Jīng*, and especially since the text is discussing a substance known (and named) for its ability to glow in the dark. I have chosen to translate the text literally, however, because all editions and quotations of this text consistently use the phrase *shénjīng* 神精 "spirit essence" here. What exactly this most subtle and refined aspect of the *shén* is, which is supported in its free unimpeded flow and communication with Heaven (*tōng* 通) by the consumption of fireflies, I leave to the reader's imagination. But it's quite a beautiful image.

58. For more details on the medical application of *yīyú*, see *Bèi Jí Qiān Jīn Yào Fāng* vol. 5 (on Pediatrics), chapter 4 on "Intrusive Upset" (*kè wù* 客忤). As a treatment for "being struck by intrusive upset in early childhood, with rigidity in the neck and imminent death," the text recommends to "take ten silverfish, pulverize them, and apply this on the mother's nipple. Make the child nurse there so that [the medicine] enters the throat. Recovery will ensue." For a translation of this entire passage, see *Venerating the Root, Part One*, p. 249. A later editorial comment adds a variation of treatment that involves massaging the child's neck and locations where the spine is rigid with the pulverized silverfish.

59. The term *xiāo* 痟 can have several different meanings. In the *Shuō Wén Jiě Zì* dictionary, it is defined as headache. In other contexts, however, it can simply refer to severe illness, or to what Wiseman translates as "dispersion thirst," 消渴, which overlaps with the modern condition of Diabetes. In the present context, however, 痟 should be read as a textual error for a rare character, 𤺊. According to the editors of the *Běncǎo Jīng Jí Zhù*, the compound 酸𤺊 refers to a feeling of weakness and soreness in the flesh.

60. More commonly referred to as *méngchóng* 虻蟲.

61. According to the *Táng Běncǎo*, the character should have a wood radical 木 on the side. All commentators agree that

this entry is placed in the section on insects by mistake but does in fact describe a tree nut. The substance is now more frequently called *fěizǐ* 榧子.

Glossary

Bandit Wind: "Bandit wind" (my literal translation of *zéi fēng* 賊風) is defined in the *Zhū Bìng Yuán Hòu Lùn*: "Bandit wind refers to the presence of racing wind that arrives from the South on the Winter Solstice, which is also called 'emptiness wind.' The arrival of this wind is able to harm people, which is why it is called 'bandit wind.' Its damage to people manifests as pain that cannot be pressed against, preventing the person from turning sides or moving, and an absence of heat in the painful spot. When the damaging wind is cold, there is deep pain in the spaces between the bones, which responds, when pressed, with bone pain. There is a sensation of deep-lying cold in the body and desire for hot things and hot compresses on the painful location…"

Barrier Repulsion: *Guāngé* 關格 is a technical term in Chinese medicine that describes a disorder now most commonly understood as vomiting above (*gé* "repulsion") and blocked defecation and urination below (*guān* "block"). In the *Zhū Bìng Yuán Hòu Lùn* (vol. 14), it is defined as "stopped defecation and urination. Stopped defecation is called 'internal block'; stopped urination is called 'external repulsion'; both urination and defecation being stopped is called 'block and repulsion'. It is due to disharmony between yīn and yáng qì and stopped flow of *yíng* provision and *wèi* defense. When yīn qì is greatly exuberant, yáng qì is unable to provision it, which is called 'internal block'. When yáng qì is greatly exuberant, yīn qì is unable to provision it, which is called 'external repulsion'. When yīn and yáng are both exuberant, they are unable to provision each other, which is called 'block and repulsion'. As a result, yīn and yáng qì form *pǐ* glomus binds, there is distention and fullness inside the abdomen, and qì is unable to move in the large and small intestine, hence causing stopped defecation and urination."

Bì Impediment: Also often called "bì syndrome" in modern TCM literature, the character bì 痺, also written 痹, is a common disease name that is defined in Sù Wèn 43 as follows: "The three qì of wind, cold, and dampness arrive mixed together and combine to form bì …. Bì means blockage (痺閉也). Blood and qì become congealed and inhibited and fail to flow. Bì can be differentiated by the three [types of] qì into wind, cold, and dampness. It can also be differentiated in bì of the skin, muscles, sinews, bones, five zàng organs, of the outside, mixed, …"For a modern TCM explanation, see the entry on "impediment" in Wiseman and Féng, Practical Dictionary of Chinese Medicine, pp. 295-6.

Bolting Piglet: According to the *Jīn Guì Yào Lüè*, "The disease of Bolting Piglet starts from the lesser abdomen, rushes up into the throat, erupts [with such vehemence that] the patient is near death, and then turns back around and stops. In all cases it is contracted following fright and fear."

Clear-Eye Blindness: According to the Zhū Bìng Yuán Hòu Lùn, the term 青盲 (there called 目青盲 "clear-eye blindness of the eye") refers to the following condition: "The eye itself does not exhibit any visible changes; the pupils and the white and black are clearly differentiated; but the person cannot see things even straight ahead. The essence qì of the five zàng and six fǔ organs must always rise to pour into the eye. If the zàng organs are vacuous and wind evil or phlegm rheum take advantage of this situation, the presence of heat results in redness of pain, while the absence of heat merely leads to the formation of internal obstruction. This means that the blood and qì of the zàng and fǔ organs fail to provide nourishment to the eyeball. Therefore the external appearance [of the eye] is no different, but the patient is unable to perceive things visually."

Center Flooding: Center Flooding is the literal translation for a gynecological condition described by Cháo

Yuánfāng 巢元方 as possibly affecting any or all of the internal organs and manifesting in heavy vaginal discharge in the associated color. The original meaning of the character 崩 is "landslide." In a broader sense here, as it is understood in contemporary TCM, it can be read as heavy vaginal bleeding.

Deep-Lying Beam: Deep-lying beam, *fúliáng* 伏梁, is a classical disease name that refers to fullness, swelling, and physical masses between the heart and the navel, due to binding stagnations of blood and qì. This condition is explained as a type of accumulation in the *Nàn Jīng* 《難經》 composed in the Hàn dynasty. *Sù Wèn* 40 describes it as "abundance in the lower abdomen… an envelope of great pus and blood residing outside the intestines and stomach, which cannot be treated."

Epilepsy: Depending on context, the term *diān* 癲, which I have here translated as "epilepsy," can have two different meanings in classical Chinese medical literature and is therefore alternately translated as "epilepsy" or "mania." Usually written in the compound *diānxián* 癲癇, it refers to epilepsy; in the compounds *diānkuáng* 癲狂 or *fēngdiān* 瘋癲, it refers to a particular type of insanity that is associated with yīn. As a third alternative, some later editions of this text and therefore also some commentators read 癲 as a textual error for *lài* 癩, meaning "leprosy." I have decided to interpret it as epilepsy for three reasons: first because of the etymology of the character includes the concept of jolting or toppling (*diān* 顛), second because some early editions actually have the character 顛 instead of 癲, and third because the compound 癲疾, as written above, is clearly defined as referring to epileptic fits in such important early classics as the *Líng Shū* (see *Líng Shū* 22).

Gǔ Toxin: The term gǔ蠱 refers to a specific type of poisoning that is executed clandestinely by people with harmful intentions. It is first attested in Shāng oracle bone inscriptions and is explained in early medical literature as a toxic concoction, prepared intentionally by placing several venomous insects in a vessel (as represented by the character) and waiting until all but one of the creatures had died. See Zhū Bìng Yuán Hòu Lùn, vol. 25, introduction. According to Donald Harper, "demonic bugs or female witchcraft are likely factors in the identity of the ailment" in the context of the Mǎwángduī manuscripts from before 168 BCE (see D. Harper, Early Chinese Medical Literature, pp. 300–301). In a later and more general sense, the term can refer to dreadful chronic and deep-lying conditions of often hidden causation that are therefore notoriously difficult to treat.

Hemorrhoids: The *Bèi Jí Qiān Jīn Yào Fāng* 備急千金要方 ("Essential Formulas Worth a Thousand in Gold to Prepare for Emergencies," comp. in 652 CE by Sūn Sīmiǎo 孫思邈) lists the five kinds of hemorrhoids as follows: "The first is called male hemorrhoids; the second, female hemorrhoids; the third, vessel/pulse hemorrhoids; the fourth, intestinal hemorrhoids; the fifth, blood hemorrhoids" (vol. 23.3).

Horse Scabies: A condition described in the *Zhū Bìng Yuán Hòu Lùn* (vol. 35) as one of the five types of scabies that is characterized by being concealed with deep roots inside the skin and by jagged eruptions, causing the sufferer to scratch without feeling pain.

Horse Toxin Entering Sores: Vol. 36 of the *Zhū Bìng Yuán Hòu Lùn* contains a section titled "Horse Toxin Entering Sores," that explains: "When people previously have sores and then ride a horse, the horse's sweat and the filth of the horse hair, as well as the horse's urine and feces, as well as sitting on the horse in a leather saddle, all of these can contain toxins. The toxic qì enters the sore, causing swelling and pain, vexation, and heat, and if the toxin enters the abdomen, it will kill the person."

Inch Whiteworm: A technical term that is most likely referring to tapeworm infestation.

Lurking Corpse: The *Zhū Bìng Yuán Hòu Lùn* vol. 23 on "The Various Symptoms of Corpse Disease" explains: "Lurking Corpse refers to a disease that can be lurking and hidden inside the person's five *zàng* organs for several years without being eliminated. Before it erupts, the body is perfectly balanced and appears as if there is no trouble at all. But if the condition becomes active, there is stabbing pain in the heart and abdomen, and intestinal fullness with panting and tension." To treat it, he includes this instruction: "Knock the teeth together two times seven times, then right away swallow qì two times seven times. Do this for three hundred rounds and then stop. Following these instructions for twenty days will make the evil qì leave. After sixty days, minor illness will be cured. After a hundred days, major illness will be eliminated, Lurking Corpse will completely be gone, and the face and body will be shining with health."

Mania: The compound *kuángyáng* 狂昜 is not found elsewhere and has been interpreted in many different ways through the centuries. *Kuáng* is a particular type of mental instability that is associated with yáng, in contrast to *diān* 癲, which is associated with yīn. Wiseman translates them as "mania" and "withdrawal," respectively, which works quite well. As Cháo Yuánfāng explains in Vol. 37 (on gynecological conditions) of the *Zhū Bìng Yuán Hòu Lùn*, *diān*-type insanity results when wind evil enters the yīn aspect, while *kuáng*-type insanity is the result of wind in the yáng aspect. In the same essay, Cháo describes the symptoms of *diān* as sudden loss of consciousness, drooling, deviated mouth, and loss of sensation in the hands and feet, while *kuáng* manifests with perverse, crazy speech, whether expressed as exaggerated self-praise or yelling or cursing, and failure to distinguish between relatives and strangers. As Cháo further explains in Volume 2 (on wind), both conditions are caused by emptiness of qì and blood, which then allow wind evil to enter the yīn or the yáng channels respectively. Outbreaks of *kuáng* mania specifically result in "desire to run, considering oneself high and worthy, or calling divine or sagely…" Concerning the second character, *yáng* 昜, in this compound, some editions of the text have *yì* 易 "change" instead, while the *Běncǎo Gāng Mù* has an obscure character composed of 易 with the dog radical instead 猲. The *Dai Kanwa Jiten* 《大漢和辭典》(Great Chinese-Japanese Dictionary," compiled by Tetsuji Morohashi and first published 1955-1960), the only dictionary where I could find this rare character, defines it as an angry dog with extended ears. Given that 昜 is in fact an older version of 陽, I have decided to read the compound *kuángyáng* 狂昜 here as referring simply to a particularly intense, rabid-like *kuáng* mania.

Pǐ Aggregations: The *Zhū Bìng Yuán Hòu Lùn* (Vol. 20 "On *Pǐ* Aggregations") describes this disease as being caused by blockage in the Triple Burner and a lack of free movement in the intestines and stomach. In such patients, excessive consumption of fluids causes these to be retained in the body instead of being eliminated. When this state is complicated by cold qì, these gather together to form *pǐ* aggregations, which are masses located on the sides of the body that hurt at certain times.

Rat Fistula: "Rat fistula" is a technical term for a disease first mentioned in the *Língshū* chapter on "Cold and Heat." There it is given by Qí Bó as an alternative name for scrofulas (*luǒ lì* 瘰癧) located in the nape and armpit. As Wáng Chōng 王充 explains in the *Lùn Héng* 《論衡》(comp. in 86 CE), since it is the nature of raccoon dogs (*lí* 狸) to eat mice, humans can consume these animals to cure this condition.

Seizures: According to the *Zhū Bìng Yuán Hòu Lùn* (vol. 45 on pediatrics), "Here are the signs for seizures in small children before they erupt, but when they are about to start: [Such patients may present with] a strong continuous and persistent fever, head shaking, and protruding tongue, or make startled tugging movements in their sleep and frequently grind their teeth. These are [the signs] that the seizures are about to erupt."

For more information on the diagnosis and treatment of seizures in small children, see the chapter on seizures in Sūn Sīmiǎo's *Bèi Jí Qiān Jīn Yào Fāng* (vol. 5, chapter 3, translated in Wilms, *Venerating the Root, Part One*, pp. 109-209). The text does mention the "120 kinds of seizures" but does not list them in detail. It does, however, offer different categories, such as yīn and yáng seizures; wind, food, and fright seizures; seizures in summer; seizures associated with milk aggregations or lurking heat; cold or heat seizures; seizures associated with the five *zàng* organs or six domestic animals; and fulminant seizures. In each case, it is of utmost importance to diagnose the specific type of seizure accurately, recognize the signs of impending attacks as early as possible, and treat accordingly.

Seven Damages: The "Seven Damages" is a phrase that is often part of the expression *wǔ láo qī shāng* 五勞七傷 ("five taxations and seven damages"), referring to debilitating conditions of emptiness taxation. In the *Zhū Bìng Yuán Hòu Lùn*, the "seven damages" are explained as food damage, anxiety damage, drinking damage (i.e., due to alcohol), bedchamber damage (i.e., due to sexual intercourse), hunger damage, taxation damage, and damage from taxation of the channel and network vessels and *yíng wèi* 營衛 (provision and defense) qì damage.

Snake Conglomeration: This is my literal translation of *shé jiǎ* 蛇瘕. This phrase is a technical term used in the *Zhū Bìng Yuán Hòu Lùn* to refer to one of the eight types of conglomerations. As described in Volume 19 on the Various Symptoms of Accumulations and Gatherings, "When a person has eaten snake but failed to digest it, a snake conglomeration is formed inside the abdomen as a result. Alternatively, the disease can be caused by essence fluids from snakes, which have inadvertently entered [the patient's] food and drink. The disease manifests with constant severe hunger but failure to move the food down when eating, blockage in the throat, and vomiting when the food arrives in the chest. The disease is located in the abdomen and appears like a snake when you palpate it."

Snake Seizures: As some research in early pediatric literature shows, "snake seizures" are not seizures that are induced by toxic snake bites, but a type of seizures that cause the body to move in a snake-like fashion. One of the methods for differentiating seizures mentioned in the chapter from the *Bèi Jí Qiān Jīn Yào Fāng* quoted above is by association with the Six Domestic Animals (*liù chù* 六畜), namely horse, cattle, goat or sheep, pig, dog, and chicken. After a description of each type based on the patient's manifestation, the text offers specific treatment advice (such as ingesting charred hooves or moxibustion locations, *Venerating the Root, Part One*, p. 214-215). Volume 11 of the *Yòuyòu Xīn Shū* 《幼幼新書》 ("New Writings on Early Childhood," compiled by Liú Fǎng 劉昉 in the early twelfth century CE), describes "snake seizures" as the seventh type of the Six Domestic Animals classification system of seizures, characterized by a "soft body, raised head, protruding tongue, and staring at people."

Spontaneous Bleeding: While *nǜ* 衄 is sometimes used in the narrower sense of nosebleed, it can also refer to any kind of spontaneous external bleeding that is not caused by external injuries, such as bleeding from the ears, teeth, or nipples. In *Líng Shū* 66, this condition is explained as being due to blood spilling to the outside as the result of damage to the yáng network vessels 『陽絡傷則血外溢，血外溢則衄血』.

Sudden Turmoil: I have chosen to translate this term literally here instead of rendering it more elegantly with the standard modern translation as "cholera." While the two conditions overlap, the understanding of "sudden turmoil" in the classical Chinese medical literature cannot be entirely equated with our contemporary understanding of "cholera." In the *Shāng Hán Lùn* 《傷寒論》, for example, it is described as simultaneous vomiting and diarrhea, accompanied by heat effusion, headache, generalized pain, and aversion to cold. In the *Zhū Bìng Yuán Hòu Lùn*, it is explained as due to a disharmony of warm and cold, as a result yīn and yáng and clear and turbid qì harass and disorder each other.

Three Worms: In the discussion on the Nine Worms in vol. 18 of the *Zhū Bìng Yuán Hòu Lùn* ("Treatise on the Sources and Signs of the Various Diseases," comp. in 610 CE by Cháo Yuánfāng 巢元方), the three [types of] worms are defined as "long worms (roundworm, ascariasis) 長蟲, red worms (a disease overlapping with intestinal flukes) 赤蟲, and pinworms 蟯蟲."

Twelve Diseases Below the Girdle: The term *dài xià* 帶下 ("below the girdle") is used in classical medical literature either as a general term to refer to gynecological conditions or more narrowly as "vaginal discharge," which is how it is generally interpreted in more contemporary literature. The "Twelve Diseases Below the Girdle" is a general expression, used to refer to the variety of female disorders that are quite literally located "below the girdle," i.e., abdominal masses, menstrual and reproductive disorders, and vaginal discharge. Táng Shènwēi 唐慎微 lists these in his commentary as red [discharge], white [discharge], clogged menstrual fluids, genital erosion, hardness of the uterus, slanted cervix, troubles and pain from sexual intercourse, lesser abdominal cold pain, blocked cervix, cold in the uterus, dreams of intercourse with ghosts, and lack of fixedness in the five *zàng* organs.

Water Disease: In volume 21 of the *Zhū Bìng Yuán Hòu Lùn*, we find the following explanation on the various types of water disease: "The diseases of water are all contracted by the *fǔ* and *zàng* organs. The formula specialists talk about them by different names, whether the 'Twenty-Four Waters' or 'Eighteen Waters' or 'Twelve

Waters' or 'Five Waters,' without clearly naming the signs. When we look for the root of the disease, it is always found in a lack of attunement between *yíng* Provision and *wèi* Defense, an obstructed and inhibited flow in the channels and vessels, and a weakness of the spleen and stomach. These factors cause water qì to spill over and scatter abundantly into the skin, causing swelling and fullness all over the body, with panting and ascent of qì, puffy swelling in the face and eyes, tension and stirring in the neck vessels, inability to sleep and rest, cold between the thighs, and inhibited urination."

Wet Spreading Sores: These sores are described in the *Zhū Bìng Yuán Hòu Lùn* as "very small when they first form, beginning with itching, then pain, and then forming sores. The fluid that emerges from them oozes out to soak through the skin, spreading gradually all over the body, thereby increasing [the affected area] bit by bit."

White Balding: A technical term used to refer to a specific disease of the scalp, described in the *Zhū Bìng Yuán Hòu Lùn* in this way: "Here are the signs of White Balding: white spots, stripes, and flakes on top of the head, initially resembling lichen, with white scales of skin on the top. Over time, itchy scabs form that turn into sores and gradually cover the entire head. When you wash and scrape the head to get rid of the scabs, there are sores with holes in the scalp that are as big as the heads of the tendons. These contain pus that oozes out, and are not painful but slightly itchy. Sometimes there are extremely tiny worms inside that are difficult to see…"

White *Lài* Leprosy: Nigel Wiseman explains the disease of "white *lài* leprosy" as "characterized by gradual whitening of areas of the skin, numbness of the limbs, heat in the joints, lack of strength in the extremities, needling pain, hoarseness of the voice, and unclear vision," and equates it with the biomedical condition tuberculoid leprosy (Wiseman, *Practical Dictionary of Chinese Medicine*, p. 675).

Wind *Féi*: The disease called *féi* 痱, or more specifically "wind *féi*" 風痱, which Wiseman translates as "disablement," is explained in the *Zhū Bìng Yuán Hòu Lùn* in this way: "There is no pain in the body, the limbs fail to contract, and the mind is not disordered. When a single arm is paralyzed, this is wind *fèi* disablement. It is treatable when the patient is sometimes able to speak. When the patient is unable to speak, it is untreatable." 風痱之狀，身體無痛，四肢不收，神智不亂，一臂不隨者，風痱也。時能言者可治，不能言者不可治。

Wind Water: As outlined in the *Jīn Guì Yào Lüè* chapter on "Water Qì," wind water refers to the internal presence of water qì that is complicated by externally contracted wind evil. Manifesting in aversion to wind and sore bones and joints in addition to puffy swelling especially in the face and upper body, it is an exterior condition.

Yīn Transmission Disease: "Yīn transmission disease" is my very literal translation of the condition *yīn yì bìng* 陰易病. In many editions, the phrase is changed to *yīn yáng bìng* 陰瘍病 "yīn ulcer/transmission disease" because it is common in early texts that the semantic component in semantic-phonetic compounds, or in most cases the so-called radical, is omitted, such as 藏 instead of 臟 for *zàng* organ. In that case, commentators have explained the character 瘍 to mean either "transmission" or "ulcer." Neither of these meanings, however, can refer to a disease that is only limited to male bodies. Instead, my decision to retain the original character is based on a passage from the *Zhū Bìng Yuán Hòu Lùn* that discusses a type of sexually transmitted disease called "yīn [or] yáng exchange" (陰陽易病). "When men have recently been cured but not yet fully healed, and women contract their disease by having sexual intercourse with them, this is called 'yáng exchange.' When women have recently been cured but

Glossary 501

not yet fully healed, and men contract their disease by having sexual intercourse with them, this is called 'yīn exchange'."

Yīn Wilt: I.e., impotence, inability to achieve or maintain a full erection. Given this context, the following phrase, "damage from severance," is likely to refer to an interrupted flow of sperm to the penis, instead of the more general meaning of severance.

Bibliography

1. Historical Sources
Arranged alphabetically by title according to Pinyin.

Bèi Jí Qiān Jīn Yào Fāng《備急千金要方》(Essential Formulas Worth a Thousand in Gold to Prepare for Emergencies). Composed by Sūn Sīmiǎo 孫思邈 in 652 CE.

Běncǎo Gāng Mù《本草綱目》(Systematic Materia Medica). Compiled by Lǐ Shízhēn 李時珍 and published in 1596.

Běncǎo Jīng Jí Zhù《本草經集註》(Edited and Annotated Classic of Materia Medica). Compiled by Táo Hóngjǐng 陶弘景 in the late fifth century CE.

Ěr Yǎ《爾雅》(Approaching Refinement). Compiled in the Warring States period by unknown authors.

Guǎng Yǎ《廣雅》(Expanded Ěryǎ). Compiled in the early third century CE by Zhāng Yī 張揖.

Jīn Guì Yào Lüè《金匱要略》(Essentials of the Golden Cabinet). Compiled by Zhāng Zhòngjǐng 張仲景 in the end of the Hàn dynasty.

Huáinánzi《淮南子》. Compiled by Liú Ān 劉安 before 139 BCE.

Huáng Dì Nèi Jīng《黃帝內經》(Inner Classic of the Yellow Emperor). Compiled by unknown authors in the later Hàn dynasty.

Líng Shū《靈樞》(Divine Pivot). Compiled in the later Hàn dynasty as part of the *Huáng Dì Nèi Jīng*.

Lùn Héng《論衡》(Balanced Discourse). Composed by Wáng Chōng 王充 in 86 CE.

Míng Yī Bié Lù《名醫別錄》(Separate Records by Famous Physicians). Compiled by Táo Hóngjǐng 陶弘景 as part of the *Běncǎo Jīng Jí Zhù* in the late fifth century CE.

Nàn Jīng《難經》(Classic of Difficulties). Compiled by unknown authors in the Hàn period.

Shén Nóng Běncǎo Jīng《神農本草經》. Compiled by unknown authors in the Hàn period.

Shuō Wén Jiě Zì《說文解字》(Explaining Graphs and Analyzing Characters). Compiled by Xǔ Shèn 許慎 in the second century CE.

Sù Wèn《素問》(Plain Questions). Compiled in the later Hàn dynasty as part of the *Huáng Dì Nèi Jīng*.

Táng Běncǎo《唐本草》(Táng Materia Medica). Also known as Xīn Xīu Běncǎo 新修本草, published in 657 to 659 by Sū Jìng 蘇敬.

Yòuyòu Xīn Shū《幼幼新書》(New Writings on Early Childhood). Compiled by Liú Fǎng 劉昉 in the early twelfth century CE.

Zhōu Lǐ《周禮》(Rites of Zhōu). First mentioned in the 2nd c. BCE but edited by Liú Xīn 劉歆 during the mid Hàn dynasty.

Zhū Bìng Yuán Hòu Lùn《諸病源候論》(Treatise on the Sources and Signs of the Various Diseases). Compiled by Cháo Yuánfāng 巢元方 in 610 CE.

2. Contemporary References Cited
Arranged alphabetically by author's last name

Anon. *Zhōnghuá Běncǎo* 中華本草 (Chinese Materia Medica). Shanghai Kexue Jishu Chubanshe, 1999.

Anon., *Zhōngyào Dà Cídiǎn* 中藥大辭典 (Great Dictionary of Chinese Medicinals). Xinwenfeng edition of 1982.

Karlgren, Bernhard, *Analytic Dictionary of Chinese and Sino-Japanese*. Dover, 1980.

Jean Lefeuvre et al., *Le Grand Dictionnaire Ricci de la Langue Chinoise* (also known as "The Grand Ricci"). Desclée de Brouwer Publishing House, 2001.

Li Shizhen, *Compendium of Materia Medica (Bencao Gangmu)*. Tr. Xiao Xiaoming, Li Zhenguo, and committee. Chinese original 1596. Foreign Languages Press, 2003.

Luó Zhúfēng 羅竹風, lead editor, *Hànyǔ Dà Cídiǎn* 漢語大辭典 (Great Dictionary of the Chinese Language). Shanghai Cishu Chubanshe, 1986-1993.

Mǎ Jìxìng 馬繼興, lead editor, *Mǎwángduī gǔ yīshū kǎoshì* 馬王堆古醫書考釋 (Philological Investigation of the Ancient Medical Texts from Mawangdui). Hunan Keji Chubanshe, 1992.

Mǎ Jìxìng 馬繼興, lead editor, *Shén Nóng Běncǎo Jīng Jí Zhù* 神農本草經輯注 (Annotated Edition of the Divine Farmer's Classic of Materia Medica). Renmin weisheng, 2000.

Mǎ Jìxìng 馬繼興, *Shén Nóng Yàoxué Wénhuà Yánjiū* 神農藥學文化研究 (Study of the Divine Farmer's Pharmaceutics). Renmin weisheng, 2012.

Morohashi Tetsuji, *Dai Kan-Wa Jiten* 大漢和辭典 (Great Chinese-Japanese Dictionary). Taishukan, first edition 1955-1960.

Read, Bernard, *Chinese Medicinal Plants from the Pen Ts'ao Kang Mu*. First published in 1900.

Rilke, Rainer Maria, *Letters to a Young Poet*. Tr. M.D. Herter. Norton, 1993.

Sivin, Nathan, *Chinese Alchemy: Preliminary Studies*. First published in 1968. Harvard University Press, 2013.

Unschuld, Paul, *Medicine in China: A History of Pharmaceutics*. University of California Press, 1986.

Wilms, Sabine, *Venerating the Root, Parts One and Two*. Happy Goat Productions, 2013 and 2015.

Wiseman, Nigel, *A Practical Dictionary of Chinese Medicine*. Paradigm Publications, 1998

Tanba no Mototane, *Zhōngguó Yī Jí Kǎo* 中國醫籍考 (Investigation of Chinese Medical Literature). Original publication 1819. Renmin weisheng: 1983

Medicinals Index – Pinyin

A

àijiǔ, 50
ānlǘzǐ, 72
ǎohuá, 258

B

bādòu, 364
bǎibèi, 45
báicǎo, 329
báiè, 402
báigé, 215
báigōngcǎo, 229
báiguāzǐ, 137
báihāo, 70
bǎihé, 196
báihuāténg, 456
báijí, 260, 332
bàijiàng, 359
báijiāngcán, 309
báijiāo, 169
báijǐngqiūyǐn, 424
báilángdú, 467
báiliǎn, 329
báimǎjīng, 295
báimáo, 455
báimù, 191, 314
báiqīng, 162
báishí, 287
bǎishí, 116
báishíyīng, 155
báishízhī, 160
báishuǐshí, 392

bǎisuìchéngzhōngmù, 272
bǎitóu, 336
báitóuwēng, 346
báitùhuò, 215
báiwēi, 360
báixiān, 209
báiyīng, 69
báiyú, 435
báiyúliáng, 153
báizhǐ, 200, 201
báizhī, 78
bǎizhī, 213
bǎizǐrén, 448
bǎizú, 432
bājǐtiān, 68
bānmáo, 429
bànxià, 315
bāshū, 364
bèichǐ, 442
bèifù, 473
bèimǔ, 198
bèizǐ, 442
biānfú, 336
biānfú, 303
biǎnqīng, 163, 451
biānxù, 343
biānzhú, 343
biéjī, 242
biējiǎ, 414
bìqīng, 450
bìshí, 386

bìxiè, 214
bǐzǐ, 443
bòmù, 248

C

cāngěrzǐ, 454
cǎohāo, 320, 466
cǎoxùduàn, 104
céngqīng, 152
cháihú, 49
cháiqī, 122
cháiyú, 86
chāngpú, 35
chángshān, 466
chángshí, 289
chāngyáng, 35
chēqiánzǐ, 52, 53
chǐjiàn, 71, 447
chímǔ, 197
chìshízhī, 158
chīxiū, 354
chìzhī, 75
chóngtái, 194
chōngwèizǐ, 46
chuānjiāo, 471, 472
chuānliànzǐ, 472
chūjī, 428
cíhuáng, 389
císhí, 286
cōngrǎn, 322
cōngshí, 276
cùjiāng, 210

D

dàdòuhuángjuǎn, 383
dàhuáng, 318
dàishēn, 232
dàizhě, 396
dàjí, 73
dàjǐ, 333
dàjiù, 374
dāncǎo, 355
dāngdào, 52
dāngguī, 186, 187
dānshā, 7, 143
dānshēn, 84
dānxióngjī, 171
dānzhī, 75
dàqīng, 451
dàshì, 319
dàyèjiīnhuācǎo, 469
dàzǎo, 130
dàzhá, 46
diānkuáng, 459, 489
diānlè, 39
dìbiē, 441
dìdǎn, 433
dìfū, 115
dìfūzǐ, 99
dìgǔ, 115
dìgǔpí, 448
dìkuí, 99, 181
dìlóu, 183
dìshēn, 197
dìsuǐ, 42
dìwén, 315
dìxīn, 212
dìxūn, 49
dìyú, 220

dōngfāngsù, 342
dōnghǎi, 449, 461
dōnghuī, 403
dōngkuízǐ, 135, 240, 456
dòufǔmù, 474
dùhéng, 447
Dùhéng, 447
dúhuó, 51
dùruò, 102
dùzhòng, 123

E

èhuī, 401
ējiāo, 170

F

fàbì, 294
fángfēng, 88
fángjǐ, 223
fángkuí, 48
fāngkuì, 320
fángmù, 121
fāngshí, 289
fāngxiāng, 201
fánshí, 147
fēilián, 440
fēilián, 95
fēilíng, 175
fēiméng, 439
féiqí, 425
fēiqīng, 95
fěizǐ, 484
fēngcháng, 416
fēngdiān, 459, 489
fēngzǐ, 7, 175

fěnxī, 395
fǔbì, 384
fǔcháng, 203
fùfán, 436
fúlíng, 117
fùpén, 132, 449
fūqīng, 391
fútù, 117
fúyì, 303
fùzhī, 189
fùzhìjiāo, 170
fùzǐ, 312

G

gāncǎo, 40, 41
gāndìhuáng, 42
gāngēn, 332
gāngqián, 202
gānguī, 186
gānjiāng, 180
gānqī, 268
gānsuì, 328
gǎoběn, 212
gégēn, 182
gèn, 312
gōngpí, 419
gǒujǐ, 213
gǒujì, 115
gǒujīng, 298
gǒuqǐ, 115
gǒuqǐgēn, 448
gōuwěn, 323, 406, 456
guādì, 278
guālóugēn, 183
guāngguì, 448

guànjié, 336
guānjié, 455
guànjūn, 331
guànlú, 331
guànqú, 336
guānzhī, 408
guànzhòng, 336
gǔcài, 69
gùhuó, 456
gūhuó, 240, 456
guǐdūyóu, 71, 103
guǐgài, 38
guǐjiǎ, 411
guǐjiàn, 265
guǐjiù, 345
guǐmù, 269, 342
guǐqīng, 212
guǐtáo, 347
guìxīn, 447
guìzhī, 111, 447
gǔyángjiǎo, 297
gùyángshí, 400

——— H ———
hǎigé, 307
hǎizǎo, 221
hámá, 412
hámálán, 93
hánshí, 397
héhuān, 266, 460
héhuānpí, 460
hēishízhī, 161
hēizhī, 76
héngshān, 326, 447
héngtáng, 238
hóngzàng, 139

hòupò, 254
hóutáo, 121
hú, 430
huáimù, 272
huáishí, 114
huájiāo, 471
huángdān, 475
huánghuán, 374, 473
huánglián, 234
huángqí, 232, 233
huángqín, 203
huángshíshí, 388
huángshízhī, 159
huángzhī, 79
huáshí, 150
huìgū, 430
huìjí, 235
huījiǎn, 476
hǔjuàn, 336
hǔlán, 222
húmá, 139
hún, 38, 77, 117, 143, 145, 261, 438
húncháng, 438
huòmǔ, 197
hùqiāngshǐzhě, 51
húwángshǐzhě, 346
húxǐ, 181
húxiè, 58
hǔxū, 225
hǔzhǎng, 316

——— J ———
jiāngshí, 291
jiǎsū, 381
jiāzhūshǐ, 259

jiégěng, 237
jiéhuá, 36
jièhuǒ, 100
jièjū, 277
jiělí, 57, 223
jiéqiāng, 422
jiěxī, 395
jílízǐ, 86
jìncǎo, 356
jīnfèi, 96
jīnfèicǎo, 321
jīngēnhuā, 96
jīngguāng, 446
jīngjiè, 473
jǐngtiān, 100
jīnzhī, 79
jīqígēn, 182
jīshǐténg, 469
jītóushí, 134
jiǔjiù, 345
jíwǎn, 61
jìxiè, 263
jīxuěcǎo, 361
jízhēn, 260
jízǐ, 313
juǎnbǎi, 81
juānfèn, 266
jùcǎo, 192
juéchuáng, 231
juéjù, 469
juélǐ, 368
juémíngzi, 94
juéxī, 345
júhuā, 36, 37
jùjùmài, 193
jūnguì, 112

júpí, 129
jùshèng, 139
júyòu, 129

———— K ————
kēdòng, 225
kōngcǎo, 198
kǒnggōng, 463
kǒnggōngniè, 290, 462
kōngqīng, 151, 450
kuǎndōnghuā, 225
kuángyáng, 469, 482, 492, 493
kǔcài, 138
kǔhù, 382
kuígé, 307
kuòyú, 423
kǔshēn, 184
kǔshí, 184

———— L ————
láncǎo, 97
làngdàngzǐ, 238
lángdú, 344, 467
lángén, 205
lángyá, 338, 467
lánhuā, 349
lánshí, 82
léishǐ, 370
léishǔ, 409
léiwán, 370
lí, 304, 494
liàn, 472
liánchónglù, 342
liǎngmiànzhēn, 460

liánjícǎo, 332
liánmù, 373
liánmǔ, 197
liánqiáo, 349, 457
liànshí, 367
liǎoshí, 275
lígài, 48
lígé, 177
líhuī, 403
lílóu, 469
lílú, 322
límǔ, 71
Líng Shū, xxv, 455, 459, 489, 497, 504
língluó, 423
língquán, 374
língshí, 85
língtiáo, 458
língxiāohuā, 458
língyángjiǎo, 299
língyóu, 62
língyú, 118
línlán, 66, 262
línshí, 144
líshí, 192
lǐshí, 288, 454
liùchùmáotíjiǎ, 406
liúgōngrǔ, 146
liǔhuā, 264
liúxù, 264
lǐyúdǎn, 305
lìzhìshí, 288, 400
lóngdǎn, 62, 63
lóngdòu, 91
lónggǔ, 166
lóngshā, 188

lóngwěi, 429
lóngxū, 104
lóngyǎn, 261
lóngzǎo, 222
lóngzhī, 77
lóngzhū, 104
lóngzǐdānyī, 419
lóngzǐyī, 419
lóugū, 430
lòulú, 92
luánhuá, 271
lùcháng, 359
lúfēngfáng, 416
lúfù, 470
lùhuò, 353
lùjiǎojiāo, 169
lùjiǔ, 224
luómó, 468
luòshí, 85
luòshǒu, 221
luǒyú, 304
lǜqīng, 477
lùróng, 296
lǚrú, 351
lǔshuǐ, 476
lútóu, 470
lǚxián, 397, 476
lùyīng, 239

———— M ————
mábó, 282
mǎdāo, 417
máfén, 7, 282, 461
máhuáng, 130, 188
màigōujiāng, 93
màiméndōng, 50

mǎjiǔ, 50
mǎlìn, 454
mǎlù, 432
mǎmùdúgōng, 345
mǎngcǎo, 369
mángxiāo, 148
mángyù, 58
mànjiāo, 270
mànjīngshí, 120
máogēn, 205
mǎshǐhāo, 227
mǎxiàn, 136
mǎxiānhāo, 227
mǎxīn, 73
mázǐ, 461
měicǎo, 40
méishí, 274
méngchóng, 483
mièxī, 73
mǐgān, 40
míhóutáo, 468
mìlà, 176
mǐwú, 83
míxián, 217
mízhī, 408
mùdān, 246
mǔdān, 224
mùěr, 458
mǔgǒuyīnjīng, 298
mǔguì, 110, 449
mǔjīngzǐ, 448
mùlán, 262
mǔlì, 177
mùméng, 438
mǔméng, 211, 455
mùmì, 54

mùxiāng, 54, 55
mùzhī, 80

——— N ———
nǎidōng, 358
níngshuǐshí, 392
niúbiǎn, 357, 470
niúhuáng, 300
niújǐ, 216
niúxī, 45
nǚluó, 267
nǚqīng, 348, 468
nǚwǎn, 228
nǚwěi, 47
nǚzhēnshí, 124

——— O ———
ǒushíjīng, 133

——— P ———
pángtōng, 86
pénglěi, 132, 449
pòxiāo, 149
púhuáng, 89
pútáo, 131

——— Q ———
qiāndān, 394, 475
qiàngēn, 208
qiānghuó, 51
qiāngláng, 422
qiángmá, 216
qiāngqīng, 51
qiángwēi, 216
qiáogēn, 243
qícǎo, 425

qǐgēn, 115
qīhāo, 330
qīngfēnshí, 400
qīnghāo, 320
qīnglánggān, 399
qīngshízhī, 157
qínguā, 195
qīngwǎn, 206
qīngxiāngzǐ, 330
qīngzhī, 77
qínjiāo, 6, 195, 256, 471, 472
qínpí, 255
qínnǚ, 50, 56, 195, 244, 471, 472
qióngjù, 333
qūcǎo, 241
quèpiáo, 348
quèwèng, 427
qúmài, 193, 454
qūrén, 86
qùshuǐ, 340

——— R ———
ráohuā, 337
rénshēn, 4, 38
rénxián, 38
ròucōngróng, 87
ròuguì, 447
rùdìjīnniú, 460
rǔgēn, 205
ruíhé, 125
ruírén, 449

S

sānggēnbáipí, 250
sāngpíxiāo, 310
sāngshàngjìshēng, 263
sānjiān, 192
sānlián, 349
shānglù, 341
shānjì, 43
shānyáng, 56
shànyú, 480
shānyù, 56
shānzhūyú, 257, 458
sháoyào, 190, 191
shāshēn, 236
shāshī, 426
shéchuángzǐ, 98
shéfú, 419
shègān, 324
shéhán, 325
shémǐ, 98
shēngmá, 106, 107
shēngtuī, 86
shèngzhēn, 321
shènhuǒ, 100
shénwū, 411
shésù, 98
shétuì, 419
shéxián, 325
shèxiāng, 301
shícán, 426
shíchángshēng, 355
shídǎn, 386
shígān, 302
shígāo, 285
shíhú, 66, 67
shíhuī, 401
shíjiǎn, 476
shǐjiāo, 270
shíliúhuáng, 7, 284
shílóngchú, 104
shílóngruì, 204
shílóngzǐ, 308
shímì, 174
shímò, 161
shínán, 269
shínǎo, 154
shíniè, 161
shīshí, 74
shǐshǒu, 93, 192
shíwéi, 226
shíxiàchángqīng, 350
shíyí, 174
shíyóu, 310
shízhōngrǔ, 146, 462
shízhū, 399
shízhūyú, 458
shǔfǎ, 302
shǔfù, 436
shǔgū, 224
shuǐhuá, 218
shuǐhuái, 184
shuǐjùn, 197
shuǐmǔhuā, 100
shuǐpíng, 218
shuǐqín, 279
shuǐshēn, 197
shuǐsū, 277, 460
shuǐxiāng, 97
shuǐxiè, 58
shuǐyín, 390
shuǐyīng, 279
shuǐyù, 315
shuǐzhì, 437
shuǐzhī, 133
shǔizhī, 137
shǔjiāo, 365, 471, 472
shǔlǐ, 376
shǔmǐ, 281, 461
shǔmò, 381
shǔqī, 327
shǔyángquán, 362
shǔyù, 56
shǔzǎo, 257
shǔzhé, 91
sīxiān, 123
sōngfáng, 113
sōnggāo, 113
sōngluó, 267
sōngzhī, 113
sōushū, 375
suānjiāng, 210
suānzǎo, 119
suī, 90
sùmǐ, 280

T

tàiyīyúliáng, 154, 450
tānggēn, 341
tánhuán, 248
táohérén, 378
tiānhuāfěn, 454
tiānlóu, 430
tiānméndōng, 39

tiānmíngjīng, 93
tiānshǔshǐ, 302
tiānxióng, 314
tiěluò, 393
tímǔ, 197
tínglì, 319
tōngcǎo, 189
tōngshí, 290
tóngyè, 372
tóngyú, 304
tóngyún, 88
tù, 44
túcǎo, 138
tǔguā, 219
tùhé, 329
tuīqīng, 391
tùlú, 44
túndiān, 407
túnluǎn, 407
tuówú, 225
tuóyújiǎ, 413
tùsīzǐ, 44
túxī, 225
tǔzhū, 56

——— W ———

wángbùliúxíng, 105
wángguā, 219
wánglián, 234
wángsūn, 229, 455
wàngyōu, 244
wànsuì, 81
wǎntóng, 263
wèimáo, 265
wèipí, 420
wēiwú, 83

wēixián, 217
wùfǎng, 173
wúgōng, 431
wúgū, 252
wūhuì, 313
wǔjiāpí, 122
wūjiǔ, 352
wūpú, 324
wūtóu, 313
wǔwèizǐ, 235
wúyí, 252
wūzéiyúgǔ, 306
wúzhūyú, 249

——— X ———

xiàkūcǎo, 358
xiāngpú, 90
xiànshí, 136
xiāoshí, 148, 449
xiǎoxīn, 65
xìcǎo, 61
xīcháncǎo, 84
xīdú, 313
xiè, 418
xiěrshí, 181
xīgōu, 358
xīmíngzǐ, 73
xìnghérén, 380
xīnshěn, 121
xīnyí, 121
xióngbái, 168
xiónghuáng, 388
xiōngqióng, 185
xióngzhī, 168
xìxīn, 64, 65
xīyí, 308

xuǎn, 138
xuáncǎo, 326
xuāncǎo, 244
xuāncǎogēn, 457
xuánfùhuā, 321
xuánhuā, 96
xuánshēn, 194
xuánshí, 286
xuántí, 464
xuánzhī, 76
xúchángqīng, 103, 469
xúchāngqíng, 469
xúchāngqīng, 350
xùdú, 344
xùduàn, 91, 104
xūwán, 396

——— Y ———

yànfáng, 173
yángcháng, 347
yángjiǔ, 50
yángqīshí, 287
yángtáo, 347, 467, 468
yángtí, 342
yángzhízhú, 339
yànhuìshí, 134
yànshǐ, 410
yáohuā, 337
yāorào, 61
yàoshígēn, 373
yázǐ, 338
yěgé, 323, 456
yèguāng, 434
yělán, 92

yěliáo, 197
yěwēng, 421
yězhàngren, 346
yì, 249, 469, 492, 501
yìmíng, 46
yìmǔ, 46
yínán, 244
yīnchénhāo, 101
yínghuǒ, 434
yíngshí, 216
yīnniè, 291, 463
yínyánghuò, 202
yīnyù, 335
yīqī, 436
yìqiáo, 349
yìyǐrén, 57
yīyú, 435, 483
yìzhì, 261
yuánhuā, 340
yuánqīng, 433
yuānwěi, 317
yuǎnzhì, 60, 61
yúliáng, 153
yùlǐrén, 368
yùmù, 263
yúnhuá, 144
yǔniè, 147
yúnmǔ, 144
yúnshā, 144
yúnshí, 230
yúnyè, 144
yúnyīng, 144
yúnzhū, 144
yúpí, 118
yùquán, 145

yùshí, 400
yùyán, 56
yǔyúliáng, 153, 450, 461
yùzhá, 145
yùzhī, 78
yùzhú, 47

——— Z ———
zàidān, 171
zàojiá, 366
zàoshè, 427
zǎoxiū, 354
zélán, 222
zéqī, 334
zéxiè, 58, 59
zhàchán, 415
zhǎngsūn, 229
zhèchóng, 441
zhégēn, 349
zhǐ, 349
zhīmǔ, 197, 236
zhǐshí, 253
zhǐxíng, 86
zhìzhǎng, 437
zhīzǐ, 246
zhōngrǔ, 462, 463
zhōumá, 106
zhú, 43
zhūlíng, 259
zhūténg, 473
zhǔtián, 328
zhúyè, 247
zǐǎo, 207
zǐbáipí, 371
zǐcǎo, 207

zǐdān, 207
zǐshēn, 211, 455
zǐshíyīng, 156, 450
zǐténg, 473
zǐwǎn, 206
zǐwēi, 258, 458
zǐzhī, 80
zuǒmiǎn, 47

Medicinals Index – Latin

────── A ──────

Achillea alpina, fruit of, 74
Achyranthes bidentata, root of, 45
Aconitum carmichaelii, processed long tuber without offshoots of, 314
Aconitum carmichaelii, processed main tuber of, 313
Aconitum carmichaelii, processed offshoots of the main tuber of 312
Aconitum ochranthum, root, stalk, and leaves of, 357
Acorus gramineus, rhizome of, 35
Actinidia chinensis, root of, 347
Adenophora tetraphylla and similar species, root of, 236
Adiantum monochlamys, whole herb of, 355
Albizzia julibrissin, bark of, 266
Alisma plantago-aquatica, rhizome of, 58
Allium fistulosum, seed of, 276
Allolobophora caliginosa trapezoides,, 424
Amaranthus mangostanus, seed of, 136
Ammophila vagabunda, 421

Ampelopsis japonica, root of, 329
Anemarrhena asphodeloides, rhizome of, 197
Angelica dahurica, root of, 201
Angelica pubescens, root and rhizome of, 51
Angelica sinensis or *polymorpha*, root of, 186
Aristolochia fangshi, root of, 223
Armadillidium vulgare, 436
Artemisia annua or *apiacea*, whole plant of, 320
Artemisia capillaris or *scoparia*, whole plant of, 101
Artemisia keiskeana, fruit of, 72
Artemisia sieversiana, whole plant of, 70
Arthraxon hispidus, whole plant of, 356
Asparagus cochinchinensis, tuber of, 39
Aster fastigiatus, whole plant or roots of, 228
Astragalus membranaceus, *mongholicus*, and other species, root of, 232
Atractylodes macrocephala, rhizome of, 43
Aucklandia lappa, root of, 54

B

Belamcanda chinensis, rhizome of, 324
Benincasa hispida, seed of, 137
Blatta orientalis, 440
Bletilla striata, rhizome of, 332
Bupleurum chinense, root of, 49

C

Caesalpinia sepiaria, seed of, 230
Calystegia sepium, flowers of, 96
Campsis grandiflora, flower of, 258
Cannabis sativa, achene of 282
Carduus crispus, whole plant or root of, 95
Carpesium abrotanoides, whole plant of, 93
Catalpa ovata, bark of, 371
Catharsius molossus, 422
Celosia argentea, seed of, 330
Centella asiatica, whole plant of, 361
Chrysanthemum x morifolium, flower of, 36
Cibotium barometz, rhizome of, 213
Cimifuga foetida, dahurica, or heracleifolia, rhizome of, 106
Cinnamomum cassia, bark of, 110
Cistanche salsa or deserticola, fleshy stalk of, 87
Citrus aurantium, unripe fruit of, 253
Citrus reticulata, peel of, 129
Citrus x wilsonii, 253
Clematis apiifolia, stalk of, 47
Cnidium monnieri, fruit of, 98
Coix lachrymae-jobi, seed kernel of, 57
Coptis chinensis, deltoidea, and other species, rhizome of, 234
Cornus officinalis, fruit of, 257
Croton tiglium, seed of, 364
Cryptotympana atrata and related species, 415
Cucumis and various species of, peduncle of, 278
Cuscuta chinensis, seed of, 44
Cynanchum atratum or c. Versicolor, root of, 360
Cynanchum paniculatum, root and rhizome of, 350
Cynanchum paniculatum, root of, 103

D

Daphne genkwa, flower of, 340
Dendrobium nobile, whole plant of, 66
Deutzia scabra,, fruit of, 375
Dianthus superbus or chinensis, whole plant of, 193
Dichroa febrifuga, foliage of, 327
Dichroa febrifuga, root of, 326

Dictamnus dasycarpus, root bark of, 209
Dimocarpus longan, fruit of, 261
Dioscorea hypoglauca, collettii, tokoro, or gracillima, rhizome of, 214
Dioscorea opposita, root of, 56
Dipsacus asper, root of, 91
Dryopteris crassirhizoma, rhizome of, 336
Dysosma versipellis, root and rhizome of, 345

——————— E ———————

Eleutherococcus gracilistylus, sessiliflorus, senticosus, heryi, or *verticillatus*, root bark of 122
Ephedra sinica, stalks of, 188
Epimedium grandiflorum, whole plant of, 202
Eriocheir sinensis, 418
Eucommia ulmoidis, bark of, 123
Eumenes pomiformis, 421
Euonymus elatus, branch or plumes of, 265
Eupatorium fortunei, whole plant of, 97
Euphorbia kansui, root of, 328
Euphorbia pekinensis, root of, 333
Eupolyphaga sinensis, 441
Euryale ferox, seed of, 134

——————— F ———————

Fejervarya limnocharis or similar species, 412
Forsythia suspensa, capsule of, 349
Fraxinus rhynchophylla and related species, bark of the trunk of, 255
Fritillaria cirrhosa, bulb of, 198

——————— G ———————

Ganoderma, fruiting body of, black, 76
Ganoderma, fruiting body of, green-blue, 77
Ganoderma, fruiting body of, purple, 80
Ganoderma, fruiting body of, red, 75
Ganoderma, fruiting body of, yellow, 79
Ganoderma, fruiting body of, white, 78
Gardenia jasminoides, fruit of,, 246
Gastrodia elata, rhizome of, 71
Gelsemium elegans, whole plant of, 323
Gentiana macrophylla, root of, 195
Gentiana scabra, root and rhizome of, 62
Gleditsia sinensis, fruit of, 366
Glycine max, sprouted seed of, 383

Glycyrrhiza uralensis, root of, 40
Gryllotalpa, 430

──────── H ────────

Hemerocallis vulva, root of, 244
Heterophylla, 223
Cinnamomum cassia, bark of, 112
Hirudo nipponica and related species, 437
Holotrichia diomphalia, 425
Huechys sanguinea, 428
Hyoscyamus niger, seed of, 238

──────── I ────────

Illicium lanceolatum, leaves of, 369
Imperata cylindrica, rhizome of, 205
Inula britannica or lunariaefolia, flowerhead of, 321
Iris pallasii, seed of, 192
Iris tectorum, rhizome of, 317

──────── J ────────

Juncus effusus, whole herb of, 104

──────── K ────────

Kochia scoparia, fruit of, 99
Koelreuteria paniculata, flower of, 271

──────── L ────────

Laccocephalum mylittae, fruit of, 370
Lagenaria siceraria var. Gourda, fruit of, 382
Leonurus heterophyllus, seed of, 46
Lepidium apetalum or descurainia sophia, seed of, 319
Lepisma saccharina, 435
Ligusticum sinense, jeholense, or tenuissimum, rhizome and root of, 212
Ligusticum wallichii, foliage and sprout of 83
Ligusticum wallichii, rhizome of, 185
Ligustrum lucidum, fruit of, 124
Lilium lancifolium, bulb of 196
Limax, 423
Lithospermum erythrorhizon, root of, 207
Luciola, 434
Lycium chinensis, bark of the root of, 115
Lycopus lucidus, foliage and stalk of, 222

──────── M ────────

Magnolia liliflora, bark of, 262
Magnolia liliflora/biondii/denudata, flower of, 121
Magnolia officinalis or biloba, bark of, 254
Malva verticillata, seed of, 135

Mauremys reevesii, syn.
 Chinemys reevesii, 411
Melia toosendan, fruit of, 367
Meloe coarctatus, 433
Monema flavescens a.k.a.
 Cnidocampa flavescens, 427
Morinda officinalis, root of, 68
Morus alba, bark of the root
 of, 250
Mylabris phalerata or cichorii,
 429

——————— N ———————

Nelumbo nucifera, seed and
 stalk of, 133
Northern snakehead fish, 304

——————— O ———————

Oenanthe javanica, whole
 plant of, 279
Opisthoplatia orientalis, 441

——————— P ———————

Paeonia lactiflora, root of, 191
Paeonia suffruticosa, bark of
 the root of, 224
Panax ginseng, root of, 38
Panicum miliaceum, seed of,
 281
Parasiticus and related
 species, 263
Paris polyphylla, rhizome of,
 354
Paris tetraphylla, rhizome of,
 229

*Patrinia villosa or p. Scabiosae-
 folia*, whole plant with roots
 of, 359
*Paulownia fortunei or p.
 Tomentosa*, leaves of, 372
Pedicularis resupinata, whole
 plant of, 227
Pelodiscus sinensis, syn. *Amyda
 sinensis*, 414
Persicaria tinctoria, fruit of, 82
Peucedanum japonicum, root
 of, 48
Phellodendron amurense, bark
 of, 248
Pheretima aspergillum,, 424
Photinia serratifolia, leaves
 of, 269
Phryganea japonica, 426
*Phyllostachys nigra and related
 species*, foliage of, 247
Physalis alkekengi, whole
 plant of, 210
Phytolacca acinosa, root of, 341
Pinellia ternata, rhizome of,
 315
Pinus massoniana, rosin of,
 113
Plantago asiatica, seed of, 52
Platycladus orientalis, seed
 of, 116
Platycodon grandiflorum, root
 of, 237
Polistes mandarinus, 416
Pollia japonica, rhizome and
 root, or whole plant of, 102
Polygala tenuifolia, root of, 61

Polygonum aviculare, whole plant of, 343
Polygonum cuspidatum, root of, 316
Polygonum hydropiper, fruit of, 275
Polyporus umbellata, fruiting body of, 259
Poncirus trifoliata, unripe fruit of, 253
Poria cocos, dried fungus of, 117
Potentilla cryptotaenia, root of, 338, 467
Potentilla kleiniana, whole plant of, 325
Prinsepia uniflora, seed of, 125
Prospirobolus joannsi, 432
Prunella vulgaris, flowering part of, 358
Prunus armeniaca, seed of, 380
Prunus japonica or p. Humilis, seed of, 368
Prunus mume, fruit of, 274
Prunus persica or p. Davidiana, seed of, 378
Pteromys momonga, 409
Pueraria lobata, root of, 182
Pulsatilla chinensis, root of, 346
Pyrola rotundifolia, whole plant of, 217
Pyrrosia lingua and other species, foliage of, 226

——— R ———

Ranunculus sceleratus, whole plant of, 204
Rehmannia glutinosa, dried root of, 42
Rhamnus davurica, fruit of, 376
Rhaponticum uniflorum, root of, 92
Rheum palmatum, tanguticum, and other species, root of, 318
Rhododendron molle, flower of, 339
Rhynchosia volubilis, leaves and stalk of, 353
Rosa multiflora, fruit of, 216
Rostellularia procumbens, whole plant of, 231
Rubia cordifolia, root of, 208
Rubia yunnanensis, 211
Rubus tephrodes, fruit of, 132
Rumex japonicus or nepalensis, root of, 342

——— S ———

Salix babylonica, flower of, 264
Salvia chinensis, whole plant of, 211
Salvia miltiorrhiza, root of, 84
Sambucus javanica, fruit of, 239
Sanguisorba officinalis, root of, 220
Saposhnikovia/ledebouriella divaricata, root of, 88, 447

Sargassum fusiforme or *pallidum*, whole plant of, 221
Schisandra chinensis, fruit of, 235
Schizonepeta tenuifolia, whole herb of 381
Scolopendra subspinipes, 431
Scrophularia ningpoensis, root of, 194
Scutellaria baicalensis and similar species, root of, 203
Sedum erythrosticum, whole plant of, 100
Selaginella tamariscina, whole plant of, 81
Senna obtusifolia, seed of, 94
Sesamum indicum, black seed of, 139
Setaria italica, seed of, 280
Skimmia reevesiana, foliage and stalk of, 335
solanum lyratum, close relative of, 362
Solanum lyratum, whole plant of, 69
Solen gouldii, 417
Solva tigrina or *walker* and related species, 438
Sonchus oleraceus, whole plant of, 138
Sophora flavescens, root of, 184
Sophora japonica, fruit of, 114
Spirodela polyrhiza, whole plant of, 218
Stachys baicalensis, whole plant of, 277

Stellera chamaejasme, root of, 344
Stenoloma chusanum, whole plant or rhizome of, 352

——————— T ———————

Tabanus bivittatus, 439
Tetradium ruticarpum, unripe fruit of, 249
Tetrapanax papyrifera, pith in the stalk of, 189
Thlaspi arvense, seed of, 73
Toxicodendron vernicifluum, dried sap of, 268
Trachelospermum jasminoides, vines and foliage of, 85
Tribulus terrestris, fruit of, 86
Trichosanthes cucumerina, fruit of, 219
Trichosanthes kirilowii, root of, 183
Tussilago farfara, flower of, 225
Typha angustata, pollen of, 89
Typha angustata, whole herb of, 90

——————— U ———————

Ulmus macrocarpa, processed fruit of, 252
Ulmus pumila, bark of, 118
Usnea longissima, whole plant of, 267

V

Vaccaria hispanica/segetalis, fruit of, 105
Veratrum nigrum, root and rhizome of, 322
Viscum coloratum or loranthus, branches and foliage of, 263
Vitex rotundifolia, fruit of, 120
Vitis vinifera, fruit of, 131

W

Wikstroemia canescens, flowers of, 337
Wisteria sinensis, flower of 374
Wolfiporia extensa, dried fungus of

X

Xanthium sibiricum, fruit of, 181

Z

Zanthoxylum bungeanum, seed capsule of, 256
Zanthoxylum bungeanum, seed capsules of 365
Zanthoxylum nitidum, root or foliage of, 270
Zingiber officinale, dried root of, 180
Ziziphus jujuba, mature fruit of, 130
Ziziphus jujuba, thorns of, 260
Ziziphus spinosa, fruit of, 119

Medicinals Index – English

A

acanthopanax bark, 122
achyranthes, 45
aconite, xxi, 312–314, 466
actinolite, 287
adzuki bean, 474
alpine yarrow fruit, 74
alum, 147
amaranth seed, 136
anemarrhena, 197
anhydrite, 289
antelope horn, 299
apricot seed, 380
arborvitae seed, 116
arsenopyrite, 400
asarum, 65, 447
ash bark, 255
Asian swamp eel, 480
atractylodes, 43
azurite, 151, 152, 163, 450, 451, 477

B

Balas ruby, 477
balloon flower, 237
bamboo, xviii, 47, 247, 474
barrenwort, 202
bat, 302, 303
bat droppings, 302
bean flowers, 384
beard-lichen, 267
bear fat, 168
beeswax, 176
birthwort, 223
bittern deposit, 397
bitter orange, 253
black and scarlet cicada, 428
blackberry lily, 324
black cicada, 415
black clay, 161
black conk, 76
black false hellebore, 322
blackfellow's bread, 370
black sesame, 139
black swallow, 360
blue vitriol, 386
bottlegourd, 382
broomcorn millet, 281, 461
bugbane, 106
bugleweed, 222
buttercup, 204, 312

C

cape jasmine, 246
carpesium, 93
carp's gallbladder, 305
cattail, 89, 90
cattail pollen, 89
cat's claw, 230
centipede (Vietnamese or jungle), 431
chain fern, 467
chalk, 402
China root, 117

Chinese anemone 346
Chinese angelica, 186
Chinese asparagus, 39
Chinese azalea, 339
Chinese blister beetle, 429
Chinese catalpa, 371
Chinese celery, 279
Chinese elder, 239
Chinese gooseberry, 347
Chinese honey locust, 366
Chinese lantern, 210
Chinese mitten crab, 418
Chinese motherwort, 46
Chinese pasqueflower, 346
Chinese sage, 211
chrysanthemum, 36
chuānxiōng lovage, 185
cinnabar, 7, 9, 75, 84, 143, 171, 207, 224, 281, 355, 390, 475
cinnamon, 110, 112, 448
cinquefoil, 325
cistanche, 87
climbing nightshade, 69
cnidium seed, 98
cocklebur, 181
coltsfoot, 225
common duckweed, 218
coptis, 234
cork tree bark, 248
costusroot, 54
cotton grass, 205
cowrie shell, 442
cow's bezoar, 300
cursed crowfoot, 204
cuttlefish bone, 306

——————— D ———————

Dahurian angelica, 201
Dahurian buckthorn, 376
deer antler glue, 169
dendrobium, 66
dianthus, 193
dichroa leaf, 327
dichroa root, 326
dictamnus, 209
dodder seed, 44
dog penis, 298
dogwood, 257
donkey hide glue, 170
dragon tree, 372
dried ginger, 180
dried soybean sprouts, 383
dung beetle, 422

——————— E ———————

earthworm, 424
elm bark, 118
elm preparation, 252
ephedra, 188
eucommia, 123
evodia, 249

——————— F ———————

fangkui peucedanum, 48
feather cockscomb, 330
feldspar, 289
fibrous gypsum, 288, 454
figwort, 194
fish poison yam, 214
flat azurite, 163
fleeceflower, 316
fluorite, 156, 450

fossil bones, 166
four-leaved paris, 229
foxnut, 134
foxtail millet, 280
fragrant thoroughwort, 97
fritillary, 198
frog, 93, 412, 464
fuzzy deutzia, 375

─────── G ───────

gaoben lovage, 212
gastrodia, 71
gentian, 62, 195
giant centipede, 431
glauberite, 392
globe thistle, 92
goat or sheep horn, 297
goji, 115
golden bell, 349
goldenrain, 271
goose fat, 173
gotu kola, 361
grape, 131
great burnet, 220
green-blue clay, 157
green-blue conk, 77
Guandong star anise, 369
gypsum, 285, 288, 454

─────── H ───────

hair, hooves, and nails from the six domestic animals, 406
halite, 476
halloysite, 450
hare's ear, 49
heal-all, 358

heartbreak grass, 323
hedgehog skin, 420
hematite, 396
hemp seed, 7, 282, 461
henbane, xxi, 238
high-grade cinnamon, 112
hijiki, 221
Himalayan Tie bush, 337
hollow azurite, 151, 450
honey, 40, 54, 174, 366
horse fly, 439
houndshark, 480
human hair, 294
humble bush cherry, 368

─────── I ───────

India pokeweed, 341
infected silkworm, 309
inverted lousewort, 227
iris, 192, 317
iron shavings, 393

─────── J ───────

Japanese apricot, 274
Japanese caddisfly, 426
Japanese catnip, 381
Japanese dwarf flying squirrel, 409
Japanese firefly, 434
Japanese hyacinth, 50
Japanese indigo, 82
Japanese or Nepalese dock, 342
Japanese peppervine, 329
Job's tears, 57
joint-head grass, 356

jujube, 119, 130, 222, 257, 260
jujube thorns, 260

--- K ---

Keiske artemisia seed, 72
kiwifruit, 468
knotgrass, 343
Korean black chafer, 425
kudzu, 182, 215, 323, 456

--- L ---

lace fern, 352, 470
lacquer, 122, 268, 327, 334, 418, 481
ladybell, 236
large-leaved gentian, 195
larger bindweed, 96
layered azurite, 152
ledebouriella, 88, 447
leech, 437
licorice, 40
lilac daphne, 340
lily, 196, 262, 324
lily magnolia, 262
limestone, 401
longan, 261
lotus seed and stalk, 133
lyreleaf nightshade, 362

--- M ---

madder, 205, 208, 211
magnolia, 121, 254, 262
malachite, 399, 477
mallow seed, 135, 240
mantis eggcase, 310
massicot, 475

meadow fleabane, 321
mercury, 143, 390
mica, 144
milkwort, 61
millipede, 432
minium, 394, 475
mole-cricket, 430
monkshood, 312–314
morinda, 68
mountain limonite, 154
moutan, 224
mugwort, 320
mulberry mistletoe, 263
multi-leafed paris, 354
multiflora rose, 216
musk-deer fragrance, 301
Mysore thorn, 230

--- N ---

native bread, 370
nephrite jade, 145
niter, 148
North China iris, 192
northern snakehead fish, 304

--- O ---

October clematis, 47
officinal magnolia bark, 254
orange day-lily, 244, 457
oriental bush cherry, 368
orpiment, 389
ostrich fern, 467
oyster shell, 177

--- P ---

pagoda tree fruit, 114

paniculate cynanchum, 103
paper wasp nest, 416
peach seed, 378
Peking spurge, 333
pennycress seed, 73
peony, 191, 246
pepperwort, 319
piglet testicles, 407
pill bug, 436
pinellia, 315
pine rosin, 113
pinkweed, 343
plantain seed, 52
potato yam, 56
potter wasp, 421
princess tree, 372
prinsepia seed, 125
privet seed, 124
pubescent angelica, 51
pupa of the nettle moth, 427
purging croton, 364
purple conk, 80
purple gromwell, 207
pyrrosia fern, 226

——————— R ———————

razor-shell clam, 417
realgar, 388, 474
red clay, 158
red conk, 75
Reeve's turtle shell, 411
refined mirabilite, 148
rehmannia, 42
rhubarb, 318
rice-paper plant, 189
royal fern, 467

rubus, 132, 449

——————— S ———————

sage, 84, 211, 446
saltpeter, 148
saposhnikovia, 88, 447
sea limonite, 153
self-heal spike, 358
shield fern, 336
shiny-leaf prickly-ash, 270
sicklepod, fetid cassia, 94
Sievers artemisia, 70
silk tree, 266
silverfish, 435, 483
single-sorus maidenhair
 fern, 355
skimmia, 335
skink, 308
skullcap, 203
sloughed snake skin, 419
slug, 423
small carpgrass, 356
smartweed, xxi, 316
snake gourd, 183, 219
snoutbean, 353
soapstone, 150
softshell turtle shell, 414
sophora, 114, 184
sour tangerine, 129
sowthistle and similar
 "bitter greens, 138
spike moss, 81
spinel, 477
stalactite, 146, 290, 291, 462,
 463
star jasmine, 85

starfruit, 467
stellera, 344
stonecrop, 100
sulfur, 7, 284
summer cypress fruit, 99
sun spurge, 334
swallow droppings, 410
sweet flag, 35
sweet wormwood, 320
Szechuan lovage, 83
Sìchuān peppercorn, 365, 472
Sìchuān prickly ash, 365

─── T ───

Taiwanese photinia, 269
talcum, 150
Tartarian aster, 206
teasel, 91
toad, 412
toosendan, 367
torreya seed, 443
tree fern, 213
trumpet creeper, 258

─── U ───

umbrella polypore, 259
unrefined mirabilite, 149
urn orchid, 332

─── V ───

vaccaria, 105
velvet deer antler, 296
venus clam, 307
vetch, 83, 216, 232, 360
Vitex fruit, 120, 448

─── W ───

wasp, 7, 175, 416, 421, 481
water betony, 277
water plantain, 58
water willow, 231
wax gourd seed, 137
weeping forsythia, 349
welted thistle, 95
white azurite, 450
white clay, 160
white conk, 78
white horse penis, 295
white lead, 395
white quartz, 155
wild snake gourd, 183
winged spindle tree, 265
wingless cockroach, 441
wintergreen (round-leaved), 217
wolfsbane, 312–314
wolfsberry, 115, 448
wood louse, 436
wood soldier-fly, 438
wormwood (redstem or capillary), 101

─── Y ───

yellow clay, 159
yellow conk, 79
yellowhead, 321
Yunnan madder, 211

Cross-Reference List for Modern Medicinal Pinyin Names

Bai Ji Li: jílízǐ, 86
Bai Jiang Cao: bàijiàng, 359
Bai Mao Gen: máogēn, 205
Bai Xian Pi: báixiān, 209
Bai Zhu: zhú, 43
Bai Zi Ren: bǎishí, 116
Cang Er Zi: xǐěrshí, 181
Chan Tui: zhàchán, 415
Chang Shan: héngshān, 326
Chong Lou: zǎoxiū, 354
Chuan Bei Mu: bèimǔ, 198
Chuan Lian Zi: liànshí, 367
Chuan Xiong: xiōngqióng, 185
Da Ye Jin Hua Cao: wūjiǔ, 352
Dai Zhe Shi: dàizhě, 396
Dan Fan: shídǎn, 386
Dan Zhu Ye: zhúyè, 247
Deng Xin Cao: shílóngchú, 104
Di Gu Pi: gǒuqǐ, 115
Di Long: báijǐngqiūyǐn, 424
Dong Gua Zi: báiguāzǐ, 137
Fei Zi: bǐzǐ, 443
Feng La: mìlà, 176
Feng Mi: shímì, 174
Fu Pen Zi: pénglěi, 132
Ge Qiao: hǎigé, 307
Gui Ban: guījiǎ, 411
Hai Piao Xiao: wūzéiyúgǔ, 306

He Huan Pi: héhuān, 266
Hei Zhi Ma: húmá, 139
Hua Jiao: shǔjiāo, 365
Huang Bai: bòmù, 248
Jiang Can: báijiāngcán, 309
Jing Da Ji: dàjǐ, 333
Jing Jie: jiǎsū, 381
Lian Zi: ǒushíjīng (seed only), 133
Liang Mian Zhen: mànjiāo, 270
Ling Zhi varieties: chìzhī, hēizhī, qīngzhī, báizhī, huángzhī, and zǐzhī, 75–80
Liu Huang: shíliúhuáng, 284
Long Dan Cao: lóngdǎn, 62
Long Yan Rou: lóngyǎn, 261
Lu Jiao Jiao: báijiāo, 169
Lu Xian Cao: wēixián, 217
Luo Shi Teng: luòshí, 85
Man Jing Zi: mànjīngshí, 120
Mang Xiao: xiāoshí, 148
Ming Fan: fánshí, 147
Mu Dan Pi: mǔdān, 224
Nu Zhen Zi: nǚzhēnshí, 124
Pei Lan: láncǎo, 97
Pu Gua: kǔhù, 382
Qian Cao Gen: qiàngēn, 208
Qian Shi: jītóushí, 134
Qing Hao: cǎohāo, 320

Rou Gui: mǔguì, 110
Rui Ren Zi: ruíhé, 125
Sang Bai Pi: sānggēnbáipí, 250
Sang Ji Sheng: sāngshàngjìshēng, 263
Sang Piao Xiao: sāngpíxiāo, 310
Shan Yao: shǔyù, 56
Shi Chang Pu: chāngpú, 35
Shu/Sheng Di Huang: gāndìhuáng, 42
Shu Yang Quan: báiyīng, 69
Song Xiang: sōngzhī, 113
Suan Zao Ren: suānzǎo, 119
Tao Ren: táohérén, 378
Tian Ma: chìjiàn, 71
Tian Xian Zi: làngdàngzǐ, 238
Ting Li Zi: tínglì, 319
Wu Mei: méishí, 274
Xian Cai: xiànshí, 136
Xin Yi Hua: xīnyí, 121
Xing Ren: xìnghérén, 380
Xu Chang Qing: shíxiàchángqīng, 350
Xuan Cao Gen: xuāncǎo, 244
Xue Yu: fàbì, 294
Yang Ti Gen: yángtí, 342
Ye Ming Sha: tiānshǔshǐ,, 282
Yu Bai Pi: yúpí, 118
Zhong Ru Shi: shízhōngrǔ, 146
Zhu Sha: dānshā, 143
Zi Bei Chi: bèizǐ, 442

General Index

A

abdominal distention, 196, 422
abortifacients, 454
absorption, 460
acute, 133, 134, 367, 471
aggregations, 31, 494
alcohol, 495
Anderson, Dr. Eugene, xxxix, xvii, 3, 455
angry qì, 177
animal(s), xix, xxxv, 2, 4, 406, 413, 464, 481, 494, 496
anxiety, 495
ascent of qì, 35, 78, 110, 146, 154, 180, 186, 188, 206, 225, 235, 247, 278, 307, 313, 323, 324, 340, 344, 356, 380, 499
ash, 255, 365, 393, 401, 403, 476, 477
aversion to wind, 36, 88, 313, 459, 501

B

bad breath, 90
bad luck, 97, 171, 259, 295, 299, 345, 348, 355, 379, 410, 451
bamboo, xviii, 47, 247, 474
bandit wind, 217, 332, 339, 396, 423, 485
barrier mechanisms, 213
barrier repulsion, 193, 294, 485
beard, 173, 263
beautiful, 6, 80, 96, 112, 243, 244, 256, 309, 378, 482
bedchamber, 495
Bèi Jí Qiān Jīn Yào Fāng 備急千金要方, 483, 490, 494, 496, 503
Běncǎo Gāng Mù 《本草綱目》, 450, 451, 457, 463, 476, 477, 492, 503
Běncǎo Jīng Jí Zhù 《神農本草經輯注》, xxxiii, 462, 471, 475, 476, 478, 480, 483, 503, 504, 506
Bernard Read, 467, 507
bì gǔ 避穀, 460
bì impediment, 6, 31, 35, 36, 39, 42, 43, 45, 52, 57, 58, 65, 66, 70, 72, 73, 86, 88, 92, 93, 98, 105, 110, 115, 116, 119, 120, 131, 134, 138, 140, 152, 155, 168, 172, 180, 182, 185, 191, 192, 195, 198, 204, 208, 209, 213, 214, 217, 219, 225, 227, 229, 238–242, 249, 254–257, 268–270, 286, 304, 313, 314, 324, 335, 339, 341, 358, 365, 366, 373, 380, 381, 383, 400, 408, 425, 440, 466, 486
biàn 變, 464

binding, 193, 326, 454
binding heat, 93, 117, 119, 206, 418
binding pain, 117, 418
binding qì, 75, 119, 125, 206, 290, 381, 418, 488
binding stagnations of blood, 488
black discoloration of the skin, 309
black spots, 44, 47, 121, 168
bladder, 48, 89
bladder qì, 99, 352
bleeding, 89, 93, 105, 171, 180, 307, 463, 497
blisters, 168, 262
blockage, 31, 81, 148, 226, 486, 493, 495
blood and qì, 36, 45, 91, 154, 169, 205, 219, 236, 254, 279, 282, 287, 296, 299, 302, 308, 346, 351, 378, 381, 412, 425, 486–488, 492
blood block, 153, 154, 169, 172, 185, 201, 203, 205, 219, 258, 306, 310, 318, 378, 395, 436–438, 441, 442
blood vessels, 25, 29, 151, 189, 279, 289, 439
bogies, 350, 374
bolting piglet, 31, 51, 380, 407, 487
boosting qì, 44, 46, 74, 96, 132, 133, 137, 140, 175, 235, 280–282, 299, 398

boosts qì, 39, 48, 56–58, 61, 68–71, 75, 76, 78–80, 84, 87, 89, 91, 92, 97, 99, 101, 110, 116, 122, 123, 125, 131, 134, 136, 138, 139, 143–146, 150, 155, 157, 161, 169, 170, 173, 174, 176, 181, 191, 196, 197, 202, 205, 207, 210, 219, 236, 241, 243, 247, 250, 251, 253, 279, 295–297, 305, 428
bound qì, 49, 50, 110, 167, 184, 221, 230, 287, 308, 316, 319, 321, 324, 329, 358, 369, 426, 427
bovine diseases, 357
brain, 102, 121, 139, 140, 154, 185, 268, 300
branches, 31, 213, 263, 310, 427
breast, 114, 146, 220, 369, 463
breast milk, 92, 146, 290
breastfeeding, 58, 86, 91, 150, 194, 222, 258, 285, 295, 380
brightens, 6, 35, 44, 49, 65, 85, 86, 90, 102, 120, 121, 125, 136, 143, 144, 146, 151, 163, 184, 193, 204, 220, 234, 243, 256, 262, 263, 266, 288, 289, 297, 303, 305, 320
brightness, 10, 46, 73, 94
brilliant, xxii, 112
bringing down the qì, 277

——————— C ———————

calming, 38, 124, 132, 244, 274, 299, 318

carapace, 481
cattle, 478, 496
cattle disease, 211
center flooding, 91, 171, 250, 258, 265, 386, 413, 487
cervix, 498
changes, xxxii, xl, xli, 31, 394, 487
channels, 11, 130, 492, 499
Cháo Yuánfāng 巢元方, 478, 492, 497, 505
charming, 303
chest, xlii, 29, 75, 93, 102, 117, 129, 155, 180, 206, 237, 241, 278, 307, 315, 326, 418, 496
chicken, 134, 182, 428, 496
child, xl, 19, 144, 308, 419, 483
childbirth complications, 430
Chinese Materia Medica, xvii, xxx, 467, 505
Chinese Medicinal Plants from the Pen Ts'ao Kang Mu, 467, 507
cholera, 31, 497
Classic of Difficulties, 488, 504
claw, 230
clear, xxi, 7, 9, 446, 462, 497
clear-eye blindness, 94, 136, 151, 297, 305, 487
cold damage, 31, 42, 91, 172, 177, 188, 198, 202, 205, 234, 250, 254, 271, 276, 291, 315, 326, 337, 364, 367, 478, 479
cold qì, 5, 17, 23, 40, 49, 52, 56, 70, 84, 96, 101, 104, 114, 115, 138, 140, 149, 150, 184, 186, 188, 192, 195, 198, 204–207, 211, 219, 221, 224, 225, 230, 234, 236, 240, 241, 243, 246, 249, 250, 254, 255, 257, 275, 278, 280, 282, 285, 287, 296, 299, 302, 306, 307, 312, 313, 316, 319, 325, 330, 334–338, 344, 356, 357, 360, 362, 384, 412, 416, 418, 427, 486, 493
cold-related, 6, 185, 212, 256
color, xxxiv, 284, 347, 450, 471, 482, 488
complexion, 6, 47, 80, 81, 85, 96, 112, 116, 137, 145, 175, 212, 256, 309, 378, 428, 482
concretions, 31, 81, 84, 86, 87, 152–154, 166, 184, 188, 221, 224, 251, 258, 287, 291, 306, 312, 317–319, 327, 328, 331, 337, 346, 358, 364, 395, 402, 411–414, 432, 433, 439–441, 476
confusion, 35, 406, 463
conglomerations, 31, 48, 51, 81, 84, 87, 93, 114, 129, 153, 154, 166, 184, 191, 198, 212, 251, 258, 287, 291, 306, 310, 312, 317–319, 328, 331, 337, 340, 341, 346, 364, 369, 378, 379, 395, 402, 411, 413, 414, 424, 433, 435–437, 439, 441, 495
connecting, 11, 91, 332, 342, 373, 460
consumption, 5, 482, 493

General Index 533

copper, 88, 151, 152, 284, 387, 390, 393
coral, 477
cosmological, xxvi, xxxviii, 446
counterflow cough, 31, 35, 48, 61, 65, 78, 83, 110, 117, 146, 153–156, 166, 180, 186, 188, 206, 209, 225, 235, 247, 249, 278, 281, 307, 312, 313, 315, 322–324, 327, 340, 344, 356, 365, 374, 380, 421
counterflow qì, 31, 35, 78, 83, 102, 110, 117, 129, 146, 154, 156, 180, 186, 188, 206, 225, 235, 247, 249, 278, 285, 307, 312, 313, 323, 324, 340, 344, 356, 374, 380, 421
cow lice, 357, 470
crab, 418, 481
crazy, 492

——— D ———

Dai Kanwa Jiten《大漢和辭典》, 493
damp itch, 98, 123
dampness, 27, 101, 104, 249, 262, 486
dào 道, 446
dead flesh, 36, 43, 65, 85, 144, 181, 209, 254, 274, 322, 332, 351, 365, 366, 388, 399–401, 408, 413, 429, 433
deafness, 31, 80, 151, 162, 172, 219, 286, 421

death, xxxii, 8, 145, 390, 483, 487
deep-lying beam, 316, 488
defecation, 31, 118, 136, 196, 211, 253, 485, 486
defense, 486, 495, 499
demonic infixation, 83, 166, 317, 323, 327, 345, 350, 364, 374, 396, 406, 407, 410, 424, 427, 429, 431, 433, 434, 442, 443
demonic qì, 83, 317, 323, 327, 332, 345, 350, 355, 374, 410, 427, 434
demons, xix, 54, 71, 265, 285, 297, 299, 301, 341, 344, 348, 378, 379, 388, 396, 406, 416, 451
dewclaw, 407, 464
diabetes, 483
diān 癲, 458, 459, 470, 488, 489, 492
diaphragm, 29, 155
diarrhea, 31, 48, 147, 150, 153, 157–159, 161, 166, 172, 176, 180, 182, 203, 228, 230, 234, 248, 281, 291, 297, 322, 384, 497
diet, 460
discharge, 31, 100, 147, 177, 227, 248, 300, 413, 420, 488, 498
disease(s), xlii, 3, 5–9, 17, 112, 115, 124, 133, 143, 145, 149, 167, 174, 194, 211, 220, 222, 232, 251, 258, 267, 278, 298,

309, 333, 337, 357, 370, 448, 470, 476, 486–488, 491, 493, 495–502, 505
disinhibiting the waterways, 97, 437
disintegrate, 454
disperse, 85, 454
disperses liquor, 220
dispersion thirst, 31, 115, 155, 172, 182, 183, 197, 219, 280, 397, 483
divine transformation, 463, 464
dog, xxvii, 213, 298, 493, 496
downward, 27, 243, 397
dribbling urinary block, 52, 76, 135, 150, 407, 410, 426, 436, 442
dried, 23, 42, 117, 180, 268, 378, 383, 473
drink, xxviii, 27, 49, 148, 186, 277, 318, 319, 324, 337, 344, 392, 495
drool, 114
drunkard's nose, 246, 262
dú 毒, xxi
dysentery, 31

――――― E ―――――

ears, 35, 56, 58, 61, 70, 90, 92, 99, 104, 116, 134, 140, 181, 262, 493, 497
earth, xxvii, xxxi, xxxiv, 5, 17, 42, 49, 115, 212, 315, 433, 441, 448, 460
East, xxii, 153, 177, 221, 284, 306, 307, 331, 358, 417, 442
Eastern, xvii, 172, 342, 364, 449, 461
eat, xxviii, 29, 461, 494
Edited and Annotated Divine Farmer's Classic of Materia Medica, 462
eliminate, 5, 17, 27, 461
emaciation, 15, 31, 205, 335
emperor, xvii, xxxii, 504
emptiness, 56, 66, 104, 139, 171, 183, 232, 250, 495
emptiness wind, 175, 247, 267, 485, 492
empty, 29, 198
enlightened, 446
enuresis, 172
epidemic pestilences, 478
epilepsy, 31, 48, 98, 262, 354, 394, 406, 407, 415, 416, 419, 422, 458, 459, 470, 488, 489
erection, 502
essence, 25, 38, 49, 73, 93, 94, 102, 112, 124, 143, 151, 279, 288, 298, 434, 446, 482, 495
essence qì, 46, 77, 80, 87, 99, 123, 132, 134, 144, 146, 150, 163, 243, 487
evil qì, 5, 6, 17, 38, 40, 49, 54, 56, 61, 62, 68, 70, 81, 83, 84, 90, 96, 100, 101, 103, 104, 106, 114, 115, 118, 119, 125, 130, 138, 140, 143, 144, 148, 149, 154, 156, 162, 174, 188, 191, 195–198, 204, 207,

211, 224–226, 229, 230, 240, 241, 246, 252, 256, 257, 261, 267, 290, 296, 308, 312, 314, 317, 324, 325, 327, 330, 332, 335–338, 345, 348, 350, 360, 366, 373–375, 378, 384, 388, 389, 392, 396, 400, 406, 407, 410, 412, 416, 418, 428, 443, 459, 491, 492, 501
exorcistic treatments, 451
Expanded Ěryǎ, 473, 503
Explaining Graphs and Analyzing Characters, 462, 504
extends the years, 35, 36, 38–40, 43, 44, 56, 58, 66, 69, 72, 75–80, 85, 89, 92, 104, 113, 116, 117, 119, 131, 133, 135, 144, 151, 153, 156–159, 161, 162, 167, 169, 177
external, 27, 471, 485–487, 497
extrudes thorns, 105
eye pain, 73, 147, 152, 163, 234, 271, 386, 398, 442
eye screens, 193, 289, 442
eyebrows, 173, 263, 401
eyes, xli, 6, 35, 36, 38, 44, 46, 49, 56, 58, 61, 65, 70, 73, 74, 77, 85, 86, 90, 92, 94, 99, 100, 102, 104, 116, 120, 121, 125, 134, 136, 140, 143, 144, 146, 151, 162, 163, 181, 184, 193, 194, 201, 204, 220, 234, 243, 244, 255, 256, 262, 263, 266, 271, 275, 276, 284, 288, 289, 295, 297–299, 303–305, 320, 328, 329, 334, 368, 382, 386, 393, 398, 425, 434, 438, 448, 499

──────── F ────────

failure of the qì to move freely, 173
fatigue, 31
fear, 19, 21, 117, 237, 487
feces, 490
féi 痱, 332, 500
female, xxxvii, 124, 228, 244, 267, 348, 489, 490, 498
fēngshuǐ 風水, 459
fertile, xxviii, 50, 387
fertility, 132, 464
fetus, 170, 172, 258, 263, 390, 409, 426, 433, 454
fetuses, 193
fire, 45, 100, 114, 203, 359, 392, 399, 434, 471
firm, 6, 40, 48, 80, 90, 115, 120, 123, 132, 135, 140, 147, 192, 256, 263, 284, 393, 400, 467
firmed qì, 221, 412
fistulas, 31, 177, 217, 232, 290, 291, 325, 344, 349, 358, 381, 388, 400, 429, 433
five slacknesses and six tightnesses, 268
five taxations, 31, 87, 250, 282, 495
five weapons, 388, 474
flat-abscesses, 69, 92, 113, 122, 157, 158, 160, 203, 216, 232, 284, 290, 325, 329, 332, 343,

344, 359, 361, 388, 393, 401, 403, 429
flavors, xxix, 5, 23
flesh, 19, 56, 74, 145, 173, 201, 216, 220, 238, 263, 295, 364, 426, 430, 483
flow, xx, xxii, 11, 25, 50, 279, 289, 295, 439, 464, 482, 486, 499, 502
flower(s), 4, 19, 36, 96, 100, 121, 144, 192, 194, 225, 230, 237, 258, 264, 271, 282, 321, 337, 339, 340, 349, 371, 372, 374, 384, 454, 457, 468, 474
fluids, 85, 130, 462, 493, 495, 498
food, 27, 31, 43, 49, 127, 129, 148, 192, 252, 273, 277, 279, 290, 318, 319, 324, 328, 337, 344, 377, 494–496
forgetfulness, 35, 61, 62, 75, 189, 234, 351
form, 7, 8, 464, 468, 475, 486, 493, 499, 500
forms, xx, 44, 193, 307, 373, 394
foul smells, 180
four limbs, 29, 45, 119, 130, 170, 181, 222, 229, 239, 242, 270, 278, 289, 332, 334, 368, 382, 411
fresh, 23, 42, 180, 268
fright, 31, 48, 166, 297, 300, 394, 406, 407, 415, 422, 423, 487, 494

fright qì, 38, 62, 83, 116, 117, 166, 174, 177, 217, 225, 236, 237, 254, 285, 296, 306, 321, 325, 356, 416, 427
fǔ 腑, 25, 40, 135, 149, 364, 487, 498
fúliáng 伏梁, 488
fullness, 84, 88, 117, 153, 175, 180, 183, 204, 210, 237, 265, 274, 286, 295, 307, 321, 328, 333, 360, 392, 425, 486, 488, 491, 499
fulminant heat, 347, 359, 360

─────── G ───────

gallbladder, 157, 298, 300, 305
gathering qì, 119, 381
gatherings, 5, 17, 31, 42, 49, 84, 86, 149, 150, 152, 163, 168, 184, 188, 194, 211, 251, 269, 288, 302, 312–314, 316–319, 327, 328, 333, 337, 344, 346, 347, 364, 379, 392, 402, 432, 437, 440, 495
generalized itching, 218, 330, 389, 399
genital, 31, 201, 251, 412
genital erosion, 122, 147, 161, 216, 272, 284, 306, 342, 354, 386, 414, 420, 498
geomancy, 459
ghost infixation, 82, 104, 215, 227
ghost(s), 27, 31, 38, 71, 82, 104, 106, 143, 171, 177, 215, 227, 230, 238, 282, 300, 342, 374, 498

goat, 56, 202, 297, 339, 342, 347, 362, 400, 467, 478, 496, 507
goiter qì, 346
goiters, 31, 221, 349, 358
gold, 79, 151, 152, 284, 321, 387, 390, 490, 503
grain, 27, 364, 460
grass, 8, 205, 207, 241, 323, 356, 477, 478
Great Chinese-Japanese Dictionary, 493, 507
Great Dictionary of Chinese Medicinals, 3, 449, 505
Greece, xxii
grows flesh, 40, 42, 86, 135, 139, 212, 253, 254, 322, 393, 397–399, 413, 414, 429, 438
gǔ toxin(s), 27, 62, 71, 82, 97, 103, 106, 175, 206, 215, 230, 259, 265, 269, 278, 289, 295, 299, 301, 317, 322, 323, 327, 333, 340, 344, 345, 348–350, 353, 364, 374, 391, 396, 397, 406, 407, 410, 416, 424, 427, 429, 431, 434, 443, 489
guāngé 關格, 485
Guǎng Yǎ《廣雅》, 473, 503
gynecological conditions, 492, 498

─────── H ───────

hair, 6, 70, 82, 173, 218, 255, 256, 263, 269, 294, 365, 406, 463, 464, 478, 490
hardness, 31, 315, 498

Harper, Dr. Donald, xxxviii
headache, 65, 185, 188, 254, 286, 462, 483, 497
heart, xxxviii, xlii, 12, 29, 70, 89, 166, 170, 244, 266, 335, 380, 413, 414, 441, 488
heart pain, 117, 122, 125, 175, 196, 260, 274, 315, 316, 331, 491
heart qì, 35, 38, 49, 50, 75, 79, 84, 90, 104, 119, 122, 125, 130, 138, 156, 158, 162, 167, 174, 175, 184, 196, 204, 207, 211, 257, 285, 297, 299, 315, 316, 428
heat, 5, 17, 27, 40, 42, 43, 45, 48, 49, 56, 62, 69, 81, 85, 87, 89, 92, 95, 96, 99–101, 113, 114, 120, 121, 129, 135, 136, 144, 147–150, 153, 166, 168, 172, 177, 182, 183, 186, 188, 189, 191, 192, 194, 195, 197, 198, 201, 203, 205, 210, 211, 214, 216, 218, 219, 223, 225, 226, 228, 230, 231, 234, 236, 241, 243, 246, 248–251, 253, 255, 257, 258, 262, 264, 274, 280, 281, 286–289, 291, 296, 300, 302, 305–307, 313, 315, 316, 318, 319, 321, 324–327, 329, 330, 334–338, 342, 344, 346, 347, 349, 351, 352, 354, 355, 357, 358, 360–362, 364, 367, 370, 371, 374–376, 379, 381, 384, 386, 388, 390, 392–394, 397, 398, 400–402, 406, 407,

412–417, 419, 422, 426, 427, 429, 433, 434, 436, 438–441, 460, 461, 468, 471, 485, 487, 491, 493, 494, 497, 500
heat strike, 47, 115, 224, 227, 254, 276, 285, 360, 448
heavenly, 5, 10, 15, 314
hemilateral withering, 173, 274
hemorrhaging, 31, 462
hemorrhoids, 31, 92, 114, 157, 158, 160, 232, 248, 284, 290, 307, 325, 338, 343, 359, 372, 388, 407, 411, 414, 416, 419, 420, 477, 490
hemp, 7, 106, 139, 188, 216, 282, 459, 461
herb, xxvii, 40, 61, 84, 90, 104, 138, 189, 192, 198, 229, 321, 326, 329, 332, 355, 358, 361, 369, 381, 455–457, 469
Hood, Dr. Brenda, xxxix
hoof, 342, 464, 478
horse, 50, 73, 136, 227, 238, 275, 295, 417, 439, 478, 490, 496
horse scabies, 264, 490
horse toxin entering sores, 490
hot, 27, 298, 400, 479, 485
hot compress, 341
hot qì, 5, 23, 192, 359, 456
huà 化, 464
Huáng Dì Nèi Jīng 《黄帝內經》, 455, 504, 505

human, xxx, xxxi, 5, 8, 10, 11, 38, 294, 425
hún 魂, 38, 77, 117, 143, 145, 261, 438
hundred diseases, 112, 124, 133, 143, 145, 149, 174, 232, 370
hundred illnesses, 228
hundred specters, 350
hundred sprites, 103, 106
hunger, 43, 50, 56, 58, 70, 74, 96, 116–118, 125, 131, 133, 134, 136, 137, 140, 145, 150, 153, 154, 157, 160, 161, 168, 173, 174, 176, 274, 276, 289, 392, 411, 495
hypertonicity, 45, 57, 65, 120, 168, 172, 173, 181, 238, 239, 312, 314, 383, 408

——————— I ———————

immortal, xxx
impotence, 98, 155, 502
inability to grasp things, 286
inauspicious, 476
inch whiteworm, 252, 458, 491
incised wounds, 31, 40, 51, 91, 105, 163, 176, 185, 186, 198, 220, 222, 276, 285, 312, 314, 323, 325, 346, 380, 386
indigo, 82, 93, 478
induce, 10, 27
inflammatory, 471
inhibited, 104, 435, 486, 499
insect bites, 31, 82, 395

insects, xxxv, 165, 293, 342, 405, 478, 479, 484, 489
interrupted pregnancy, 395, 476
intestinal, 48, 248, 353, 407, 416, 419, 490, 491
intestinal afflux, 150, 157, 159, 161, 180, 203, 230, 234, 322
intestinal flukes, 275, 498
intestinal rumbling, 228, 315
intrusive upset, 483
itching, 46, 253, 262, 499
itchy, 113, 320, 322, 338, 342, 343, 359, 362, 369, 390, 399, 401, 403, 500

J

Japanese, xxx, 50, 82, 274, 312, 329, 342, 381, 409, 426, 434
jaundice, 31, 43, 101, 157, 159, 184, 203, 207–209, 248, 264, 479
jī guān 機關, 455
jīng essence, 235, 457
joints, 65, 80, 88, 95, 98, 110, 146, 152, 177, 189, 195, 204, 214, 216, 222, 252, 269, 286, 320, 335, 365, 455, 459, 500, 501
joy, xxvii, 79
joyful, 244, 303

K

kidney qì, 76, 161, 194, 269, 280

kill, 19, 21, 249, 269, 378, 379, 479, 491
killing grain, 277, 460
knees, 45, 134, 229, 239, 455
knife, 8, 237, 417
knotted flesh, 47
kuáng mania, 300, 346, 360, 367, 397, 406, 469, 492, 493
kuángyáng 狂易, 469, 482, 492, 493

L

lack of joy, 351, 353
lacquer, 122, 268, 327, 334, 418, 481
lactation, 198
lameness, 122
larynx, 324
lead, 151, 394, 395, 475, 476, 506
leave(s), 10, 31, 61, 130, 140, 192, 238, 247, 250, 264, 269, 353, 357, 369, 371, 372, 446, 473, 477, 478, 481, 482, 491
Leo Lok, xxxix, 446, 451, 455, 461
leprosy, 232, 401, 459, 489, 500
Lǐ Shízhēn 李時珍, 450, 457, 463, 466, 476, 477, 503
light, xlii, 6, 10, 11, 95, 303, 446, 450, 463, 466, 473
lightening, 9, 100, 175, 244, 478
lingering heat, 72, 320
liquor, 23, 218, 420, 481
liquor blisters, 246

liù chù 六畜, 496
liver, 284, 302, 468
liver qì, 77, 157
long-term consumption, 6, 9, 451
longevity, xxix, 5, 105, 140, 240, 387, 460
love, xxvi, xxxvii, 12, 50, 482
lower, xxxi, xxxv, 5, 17, 95, 299, 311, 363, 377, 385, 405, 456, 465, 488
lumbar pain, 123, 169, 170, 263, 310, 353
lumbus, 134, 213, 214, 231, 420, 455
Lùn Héng 《論衡》, 493, 504
lung qì, 78, 160, 236
lurking corpse, 39, 395, 424, 443, 491
lurking intestines, 407, 476

———— M ————

maggots, 477
male, 224, 244, 314, 490, 501
malign qì, 71, 98, 100, 103, 214, 220, 247, 274, 277, 290, 295, 296, 299, 301, 323, 338, 344, 345, 348, 350, 351, 355, 362, 388, 393, 396, 401, 425
malign worms, 189, 247, 297, 351, 362, 378, 388, 389
mange qì, 356, 362, 393
mania, 458, 469, 482, 488, 492
marrow, 29, 39, 42, 48, 139, 140, 157, 158, 160, 268, 300, 373

Mǎwángduī Gǔ Yīshū Kǎoshì 《馬王堆古醫書考釋》, 467, 506
measles, 253
measures, 17
meat, xxviii, 215
medicinal bath, 46, 231, 357, 375
menstrual, 11, 219, 306, 402, 425, 436, 437, 498
mercury, 143, 390
metal, 96
middle, xxi, xxxi, xxxv, 5, 15, 52, 136, 179, 245, 255, 273, 283, 293, 453
mind, 4, 9–11, 455, 500
Míng Yī Bié Lù 《名醫別錄》, xxxiv, 446, 461, 477, 504
miscarriage(s), 45, 476
moles, 274, 401, 403
mother, xxxix, 19, 46, 71, 100, 144, 197, 198, 236, 483
mouth, xxi, 78, 85, 90, 117, 285, 325, 330, 492
move, xl, 10, 11, 47, 48, 85, 247, 486, 495, 496
movement, 27, 31, 397, 493
moves down qì, 57, 66, 121, 129, 197, 218, 247, 249, 274, 275, 277, 282, 308, 315, 321, 365, 380, 381, 394
moxibustion, 479, 496
mushroom, 133, 137, 331, 466, 472

———— N ————

nail, 478

General Index   541

nails, xxv, 406, 478
nán hǎi 南海, 480
Nàn Jīng 《難經》, 488, 504
nǎohù 腦戶, 102
nasal congestion, 125
Nathan Sivin, 475, 507
native, xxvii, 181, 183, 197, 212, 219, 220, 370, 468
navel, 488
neck, 221, 349, 435, 455, 483, 499
Nichter, Dr. Mark, xxxviii
night, 29, 309, 415, 434, 464
night-vision, 303
nightmares, 54, 299, 301, 406
nine orifices, 35, 61, 65, 76, 120, 130, 146, 151, 152, 162, 189, 207, 211, 290, 366, 439
nine radiances, 394
nine worms, 120, 497
nine-fold-radiance, 475
nipples, 497
nurturing, xxix, 5, 15, 124
nurturing the qì, 133, 157–161, 280
nutrients, 460

——————— O ———————

obliviousness, 360
obstructed, 464, 499
ointment, 201
old, xxxii, 23, 49, 106, 146, 148, 166, 290, 318, 346, 350, 375, 431
older, 19, 469, 472, 493
older people, 213

oozes, 499, 500
open sores, 275, 353, 356, 393

——————— P ———————

palpitation qì, 217, 254
palpitations, 38, 116, 117, 237, 297, 302, 321, 356
panting, 225, 252, 285, 307, 340, 356, 491, 499
papules, 46
paralyzed, 500
patient(s), xxxix, 7, 12, 25, 182, 231, 471, 479, 487, 493–496, 500
patterns, xxvii, 307, 315
pediatric, 464, 496
penis, 68, 87, 202, 287, 295, 298, 299, 384, 446, 502
pepper, 6, 256, 365
perspicacity, 76, 138
pharynx, 324, 340
Philological Investigation of the Ancient Medical Texts from Mawangdui, 467, 506
phlegm, 326, 487
physical trauma, 468
pǐ aggregations, 149, 337, 364, 400, 493
pǐ glomus, 327, 414, 439, 486
pig, 192, 259, 270, 496
pills, 23, 456
pinworms, 477, 498
plump, 282
plump and healthy, 44, 58, 71, 124, 131, 279, 295
pò 魄, 38, 78, 117, 143, 145, 261

poisoning, xxviii, 31, 215, 391, 406, 489
poisonous, xxi, 5, 389, 479
poison(s), xxi, xxix, 82, 83, 214, 313, 331, 344, 345
polyps, 401, 403, 414, 432
powders, 23
Practical Dictionary of Chinese Medicine, 486, 500, 507
premature death, 106
propagates children, 87
protruding tongue, 217, 354, 494, 496
provision, 486, 495, 499
puffy swelling, 222, 275, 278, 304, 328, 334, 368, 382, 459, 499, 501
pulse, 202, 250, 490
pupils, 446, 487
pus, 159, 166, 176, 232, 264, 351, 383, 488, 500
putrefaction, 45, 90, 276, 291

─────── Q ───────

qì
  angry qì, 177
  ascent of qì, 35, 78, 110, 146, 154, 180, 186, 188, 206, 225, 235, 247, 272, 278, 307, 313, 323, 324, 340, 344, 356, 380, 4994
  bladder qì, 352
  blood and qì, 36, 45, 154, 236, 254, 282, 296, 302, 346, 351, 378, 381, 425, 486–488, 492
  boosting qì, 44, 74, 96, 132, 133, 137, 140, 175, 235, 280–282, 299, 398
  boosts qì, 39, 48, 56–58, 61, 68–71, 75, 76, 78–80, 84, 87, 89, 91, 92, 97, 99, 101, 110, 116, 122, 123, 125, 131, 134, 136, 138, 139, 143–146, 150, 155, 157, 161, 169, 170, 173, 174, 176, 181, 191, 196, 197, 202, 205, 207, 210, 219, 236, 241, 243, 247, 250, 251, 253, 279, 295–297, 305
  bound qì, 49, 50, 110, 167, 184, 221, 230, 287, 308, 316, 319, 321, 324, 329, 358, 369, 426, 427
  bringing down the qì, 277
  cold qì, 5, 17, 23, 40, 49, 52, 56, 84, 96, 101, 104, 114, 115, 138, 140, 149, 184, 186, 188, 192, 195, 206, 207, 211, 219, 221, 224, 225, 234, 236, 240, 241, 243, 249, 254, 255, 257, 275, 278, 280, 282, 285, 287, 302, 306, 312, 316, 319, 325, 330, 335–338, 356, 357, 360, 384, 412, 416, 418, 427, 486, 493
  counterflow qì, 31, 35, 78, 83, 102, 110, 117, 129, 146, 154, 156, 180, 186, 188, 206, 225, 235, 247, 249, 278, 285,

307, 312, 313, 323, 324, 340, 344, 356, 380, 421
demonic qì, 317, 323, 327, 332, 355, 427, 434
essence qì, 46, 77, 80, 87, 99, 123, 132, 134, 146, 150, 163, 487
evil qì, 5, 6, 17, 38, 40, 49, 54, 56, 61, 62, 68, 70, 81, 83, 84, 90, 96, 100, 101, 103, 104, 106, 114, 115, 118, 119, 125, 130, 138, 140, 144, 148, 149, 154, 156, 162, 174, 188, 191, 195–198, 204, 207, 211, 224–226, 229, 230, 240, 241, 246, 252, 256, 257, 261, 267, 290, 296, 308, 312, 314, 317, 324, 325, 327, 330, 332, 335–338, 345, 348, 350, 360, 366, 373–375, 378, 384, 388, 389, 392, 396, 400, 406, 407, 410, 412, 416, 418, 428, 443, 491
failure of the qì to move freely, 173
firmed qì, 221, 412
fright qì, 38, 62, 83, 166, 177, 217, 225, 236, 237, 254, 285, 296, 306, 321, 325, 356
gathering qì, 119, 381
goiter qì, 221, 346, 358
heart qì, 50, 75, 79, 84, 104, 119, 122, 125, 130, 138, 156, 158, 162, 167, 174, 184, 196, 204, 207, 211, 257, 285, 297, 299, 315, 316, 428

hot qì, 23, 192, 359, 456
kidney qì, 76, 161, 194, 269, 280
liver qì, 77, 157
lung qì, 78, 160, 236
mange qì, 362, 393
malign qì, 71, 100, 103, 220, 247, 277, 290, 295, 296, 301, 338, 344, 345, 348, 350, 362, 388, 401, 425
moves down qì, 57, 66, 121, 129, 197, 218, 247, 249, 274, 275, 277, 282, 308, 315, 321, 365, 380, 381, 394
nurturing the qì, 133, 157–161
palpitation qì, 217, 254
perspicacity, 76, 138
of fright, 62, 130, 174, 224, 225, 228, 236, 237, 295, 302, 321, 325, 329, 354, 356, 419
of mange and scabies, 393
of open sores, 353, 356
qí Bó, xxxii, 493
qì of the zàng 臟, 140, 487
red qì, 158, 359, 396
reversal qì, 270
spleen qì, 79, 159, 280
stomach qì, 49, 130, 150, 192, 246, 280, 332, 370, 499, 525, 528
sweat qì, 220, 267
toxic qì, 163, 191, 243, 256, 269, 278, 317, 321, 335, 336, 338, 370, 387, 412, 418, 428, 443, 491

544　　神農本草經 *Shén Nóng Běncǎo Jīng*

unclogs the qì, 76, 78, 130, 207, 211, 408
yīn qì, 68, 71, 87, 161, 182, 243, 332, 334, 486
Qín, 50, 56, 195, 244, 471, 472
quieting the fetus, 169

───── R ─────

radiance, 446, 475
rale in the throat, 340
rat fistula, 493
red qì, 158, 359, 396
refined, xxx, 147–149, 153, 482
reflux, 394
reproductive disorders, 498
rest, xl, 209, 499
restless sleep, 488
retching, 31, 110, 182
reversal qì, 270
rheum, 31, 318, 328, 487
rhinoceros horn, 478
rib-sides, 102, 117, 237, 241, 321, 425
Rihui, Dr. Long, xxxix
roosters, 451
roundworm, 466, 498
ruler, 19, 328, 446

───── S ─────

sage, 84, 211, 446
salt, 149, 397, 398, 476
scabies, 113, 320, 322, 338, 342, 343, 356, 359, 362, 367, 369, 389, 390, 399, 401, 403, 413, 490
scalp, 499, 500
scrofula, 349, 353, 358, 376, 381
seizures, 51, 62, 166, 167, 172, 174, 198, 217, 223–225, 228, 294–296, 300, 301, 309, 329, 354, 386, 394, 406, 407, 415, 416, 419, 422, 423, 427, 436, 464, 494, 496
sense, xvii, 2, 10, 446, 463, 464, 466, 470, 471, 478, 480, 481, 488, 490, 496
Separate Records by Famous Physicians, xxxiv, 446, 504
seven damages, 31, 87, 220, 282, 495
severance, 44, 50, 62, 114, 176, 183, 202, 268, 295, 373, 502
sexual intercourse, 482, 495, 498, 502
shàn-type (mounding), 48, 51, 122, 191, 198, 212, 310, 328, 340, 341, 369, 435
Shāng Hán Lùn 《傷寒論》, 497
sharpening intelligence, 74
shé jiǎ 蛇瘕, 495
sheep, 50, 297, 342, 347, 362, 400, 467, 478, 496
shortness of breath, 50, 239, 340
Shuō Wén Jiě Zì 《說文解字》, 11, 462, 480, 483, 504
signs, 31, 494, 495, 497, 499, 505
six domestic animals, 406, 494, 496
sleep, xxvii, 138, 494, 499

snake, 98, 183, 219, 354, 419, 424, 431, 481
snake bite(s), 31, 331, 406, 443, 496
snake conglomeration, 495
snake seizures, 325, 419, 496
snivel, 102
soil, xxviii, 50, 104, 370, 423, 476
solid, xxvi, xl, 129, 138, 328
South China Sea, 480
southern, xxi, xxv, 408, 447, 449, 472
southern miasmic qì, 406, 478
spine, 134, 213, 231, 263, 483
spirit illumination, 6, 9–11, 83, 97, 110, 129, 143, 162, 167, 171, 180, 230, 238, 247, 256, 261, 263, 277, 282, 394, 451, 482
spirit immortal, 75–79, 89, 134, 149, 154, 387, 388, 390
spittle, 114
spleen, 189
spleen qì, 79, 130, 159, 280, 499
spontaneous bleeding, 222, 496, 497
spotting, 91, 462
sprains, 31
static blood, 72, 89, 93, 205, 219, 224, 291, 300, 318, 378, 381, 437–439
stomach, 29, 50, 66, 138, 148, 189, 224, 248, 280, 288, 318, 394, 398, 460, 488, 493
stomach qì, 49, 130, 150, 192, 246, 280, 332, 370, 499
stone strangury, 308, 386, 417, 426, 429
stones, xxxv, 19, 423
strangury, 104, 198, 209, 310, 468
strength, 40, 44, 56, 58, 61, 71, 89, 91, 103, 131–133, 136, 139, 202, 238, 500
strengthening, xx, 132, 161, 235
Sù Wèn 《素問》, 446, 448, 455, 486, 488, 505
sudden turmoil, 228, 281, 497
summer-heat, 145, 154
Sūn Sīmiǎo 孫思邈, xxxvii, xxxix, 471, 490, 494, 503
supplementing the center, 124, 133, 276, 281, 282
suppurating sores, 222
sweat, 130, 250, 313, 490
sweat qì, 220, 267
sweating, 43, 180, 188, 265, 276, 315, 421, 456
Systematic Materia Medica, 450, 503

——————— T ———————

Tàiyīn, 478
Táng Shènwēi 唐慎微, 498
Táo Hóngjǐng 陶弘景, xxix, xxxi, xxxiii, xxxv, xxxvi, 446, 448, 450, 455–457, 462, 466, 468, 469, 474, 475, 477, 481, 503, 504

taxation(s), 31, 66, 87, 170, 205, 226, 235, 250, 282, 495
tearing, 36, 73, 94, 102, 125, 184, 201, 234, 271, 366, 438
teeth, 6, 90, 120, 147, 166, 256, 263, 296, 362, 368, 491, 494, 497
tension, 114, 212, 247, 333, 491, 499
tetany, 43, 51, 167, 172, 174, 224, 247, 294, 300, 301, 323, 386, 406, 436, 464
thighs, 499
thirst, 93, 145, 247, 281, 461
three [types of] worms, 39, 57, 83, 162, 249, 252, 254, 257, 288, 289, 301, 309, 317, 330, 336, 343, 354, 367, 370–372, 395, 424, 431, 443, 497
throat, 31, 85, 86, 110, 192, 198, 225, 315, 380, 430, 440, 466, 483, 487, 496
tigers, 297
tin mirror knobs, 395
tongue, 85, 117, 285
toothache, 31
toxic qì, 163, 191, 243, 249, 256, 269, 278, 312, 316, 317, 321, 324, 335, 336, 338, 340, 344, 348, 350, 366, 370, 380, 387, 412, 418, 425, 428, 443, 491
transcendence, xxxiii, 451, 464
transform, 8, 143, 149, 151, 152, 284, 290, 387, 424, 464

Treatise on the Sources and Signs of the Various Diseases, 497, 505
triple burner, 493
tumors, 27, 221, 349
twelve diseases below the girdle, 220, 298, 498

——————— U ———————

ulcer, 501
unclogs the qì, 76, 78, 130, 207, 211, 408
urinary block, 104
urination, 31, 104, 118, 136, 158, 184, 191, 193, 195, 196, 202, 205, 211, 223, 280, 289, 294, 308, 310, 352, 367, 368, 375, 410, 435, 468, 485, 486, 499
urine, 48, 52, 89, 93, 96, 99, 117, 123, 135, 150, 226, 490
uterus, 114, 156, 287, 462, 498

——————— V ———————

vacuity, 15, 31, 205, 272
vacuous, 25, 487
vaginal, 31, 147, 177, 186, 227, 248, 250, 420, 462, 488, 498
vaginal bleeding, 170, 265, 279, 300, 386, 413, 488
vaginal spotting, 100, 154, 166, 171, 201, 251, 272, 287, 296, 306, 396, 402, 411, 417
vertex, 407, 470
vexation, 84, 88, 93, 100, 117, 153, 183, 198, 204, 210, 274,

281, 286, 288, 307, 367, 392, 397, 461, 488, 491
voice, 35, 500
vomiting, 27, 31, 110, 162, 182, 278, 326, 333, 394, 397, 398, 485, 496, 497

W

Wáng Chōng 王充, 493, 504
warm malaria, 31, 48, 103, 177, 186, 188, 223, 301, 326, 329, 337, 339, 346, 348, 360, 364, 431
Warring States, 471, 503
warts, 310, 403
wasp, 7, 175, 416, 421, 481
water disease, 333, 337, 498
water qì, 46, 58, 72, 184, 197, 218, 275, 278, 321, 323, 334, 344, 459, 499, 501
wèi 味, 5
welling-abscesses, 27, 31, 85, 91, 113, 163, 175, 184, 193, 217, 221, 222, 224, 260, 264, 275, 296, 302, 329, 332, 340, 341, 349, 353, 369, 383, 399, 407, 408, 412, 430, 454
west, xxii, 258, 471, 472
western, xxi, xxiii, xl, 4, 12, 181, 257, 327, 362, 365, 398, 472
wet spreading sores, 343, 361, 499
white, 69, 78, 82, 100, 120, 137, 153, 155, 158, 160, 162, 168, 169, 172, 177, 191, 192, 201, 209, 215, 229, 248, 250, 251, 255, 260, 284, 287, 295, 306, 314, 329, 331, 332, 360, 371, 392, 395, 402, 411, 417, 420, 425, 435, 447, 450, 466, 467, 472, 487, 498, 499
white balding, 113, 168, 356, 390, 399, 432, 499
white lài leprosy, 246, 500
white soaking, 147, 171, 272
Wilms, Dr. Sabine PhD, xxiii, xxv, xxxvii, 494, 507
wilting reversal, 206
wind, 6, 27, 35, 43, 51, 58, 68, 70, 72, 85, 88, 101, 102, 104, 113, 131, 140, 144, 152, 156, 172, 180, 192, 198, 201, 204, 209, 214, 223, 228, 232, 240, 242, 249, 253, 255, 256, 262, 268, 270, 312, 314, 330, 351, 366, 369, 393, 408, 459, 485–487, 492, 494, 500
Wind Féi, 332, 500
wind head pain, 88, 121, 181, 212
wind strike, 31, 47, 185, 188, 222, 224, 227, 254, 276, 285, 313, 333, 360, 435, 448
wind water, 222, 264, 275, 323, 347, 459, 501
wisdom, xxxix, 38, 61, 62, 75, 158
Wiseman, Dr. Nigel, xxxviii, 500, 507
withdrawal, 167, 470, 492

withstand aging, 6, 36, 45, 51, 52, 62, 90, 93, 99, 101, 105, 120, 121, 123, 133, 134, 137, 138, 173, 176, 256, 259, 268, 276, 277
wolves, 297
women, 31, 51, 81, 87, 91, 98, 100, 114, 150, 156, 166, 169–171, 177, 185, 186, 194, 201, 209, 212, 220, 227, 234, 248, 251, 258, 265, 267, 272, 279, 284, 298, 300, 306, 310, 329, 342, 353, 370, 386, 395, 396, 402, 413, 435, 436, 462, 502
wounds, 100, 114, 216, 351, 389, 391, 471
wǔ láo qī shāng 五勞七傷, 495

————— Y —————

yáng, 19, 35, 149, 287, 458, 464, 467, 469, 479, 486, 492, 494, 497
yáng exchange, 501, 502
Yellow Emperor's Inner Classic, 455
yīn, 19, 66, 459, 463, 464, 479, 486, 489, 492, 494
yīn essence, 87, 235, 243, 310, 428, 457
yīn exchange, 309, 501, 502
yīn jīng 陰精, 235, 457
yīn qì, 68, 71, 87, 161, 182, 235, 243, 269, 287, 332, 334, 428, 486, 497
yīn transmission disease, 501
yīn wilt, 68, 98, 155, 202, 239, 287, 298, 310, 428, 502
yīn yáng bìng 陰陽病, 501
yīn yì bìng 陰易病, 501
yíng wèi 營衛, 486, 495, 499

————— Z —————

zàng 臟 organs, 25, 35, 38, 40, 58, 62, 66, 68, 70, 72, 73, 81, 87, 90, 113–116, 119, 121, 124, 132, 135, 138–140, 143–146, 148, 168, 174, 206, 224, 229, 244, 248, 253, 261, 266, 268, 282, 318, 321, 335, 364, 374, 486, 487, 491, 494, 498
zhāng yī 張揖, 473, 503
zhēn bird, 406, 479
Zhōnghuá Běncǎo《中華本草》, 467, 505
Zhōngyào Dà Cídiǎn《中藥大辭典》, 3, 449, 455, 468–470, 473, 505

Lightning Source UK Ltd.
Milton Keynes UK
UKHW011312180221
378997UK00003B/412